HEALTHCARE ADMINISTRATOR SPECIALTY CROSSWORDS

A FUN AND EFFECTIVE APPROACH
TO STUDYING FOR LICENSURE EXAMS

BY: HELENE MOLNAR, LNHA, MHA

Cover design and illustration by Helene V. Molnar
Book design and text composition by Helene V. Molnar

ISBN-13: 978-1514871362

ISBN-10: 151487136X

ALSO BY AUTHOR:

Nursing Specialty Crosswords: A Fun and Effective Approach to Studying for Licensure Exams.

DEDICATION:

This book is dedicated to my parents, Ed and Carol, both retired healthcare professionals who provided the highest quality of care throughout their careers and encouraged me to do the same. And to my children, Victoria and Justyn, who inspire me daily, and whom I love with all of my heart.

PUZZLE # 1

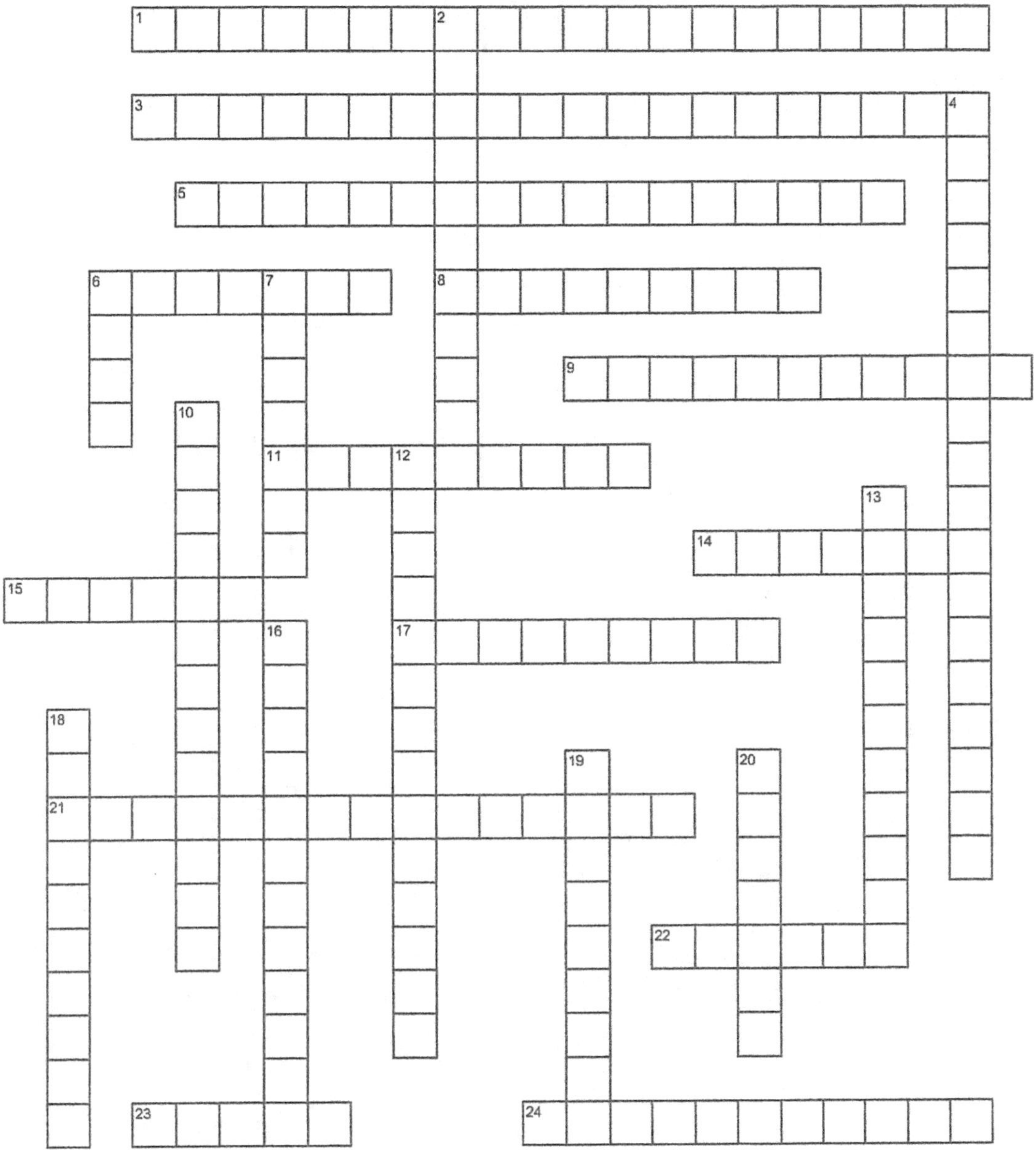

ACROSS

1 To attach metal disks to one's scalp to measure electrical activity in the brain. Used for epilepsy and other brain disorders
3 Often the largest source of deductions from revenue in NF's. (2 wds)
5 M.R. (2 wds)
6 This department must be staffed for twelve or more hours per day/ evening, in a 24-hour period
8 h.s. (2 wds)
9 F.A.D. (3 wds)
11 A disease caused by the loss of elasticity in lung tissues, which causes a build-up of carbon dioxide
14 Dies with a will
15 A request for a higher court to review a lower courts decision
17 A quality indicator that provides a description of what took place with a resident over the course of the past two MDS's or OASIS assessments
21 His theory states that aging occurs because of a limit of about fifty divisions for certain key groups of cells in humans (2 wds)
22 The result or product of one's work
23 Written defamation of character
24 This condition is difficult to diagnose, and symptoms may be similar to those of a minor stroke

DOWN

2 Any incidental by-product(s) associated with a particular course of action
4 When a business is owned by one person (2 wds)
6 In dietary, this type of schedule is retained for thirty days
7 Symptoms of this disorder may include fantasizing, avoiding eye contact, fidgeting, insomnia, and isolation from others
10 M.I. (2 wds)
12 Herzberg stated that these do not motivate employees, but are still essential to maintaining satisfaction. They are considered the most minimally acceptable work conditions. An example is satisfactory wages/ benefits (2 wds)
13 The legal process when a plaintiff obtains goods or money belonging to the defendant, held by a third party, what are (or will be) due to the plaintiff
16 When one's blood pressure is above 160/95.
18 When the presence or absence of one job behavior effects ones entire performance evaluation (2 wds)
19 The ability of current assets to meet current liabilities. The ability to easily obtain cash from assets.
20 When something destroys tissue by local application, it is said to be this.

PUZZLE # 2

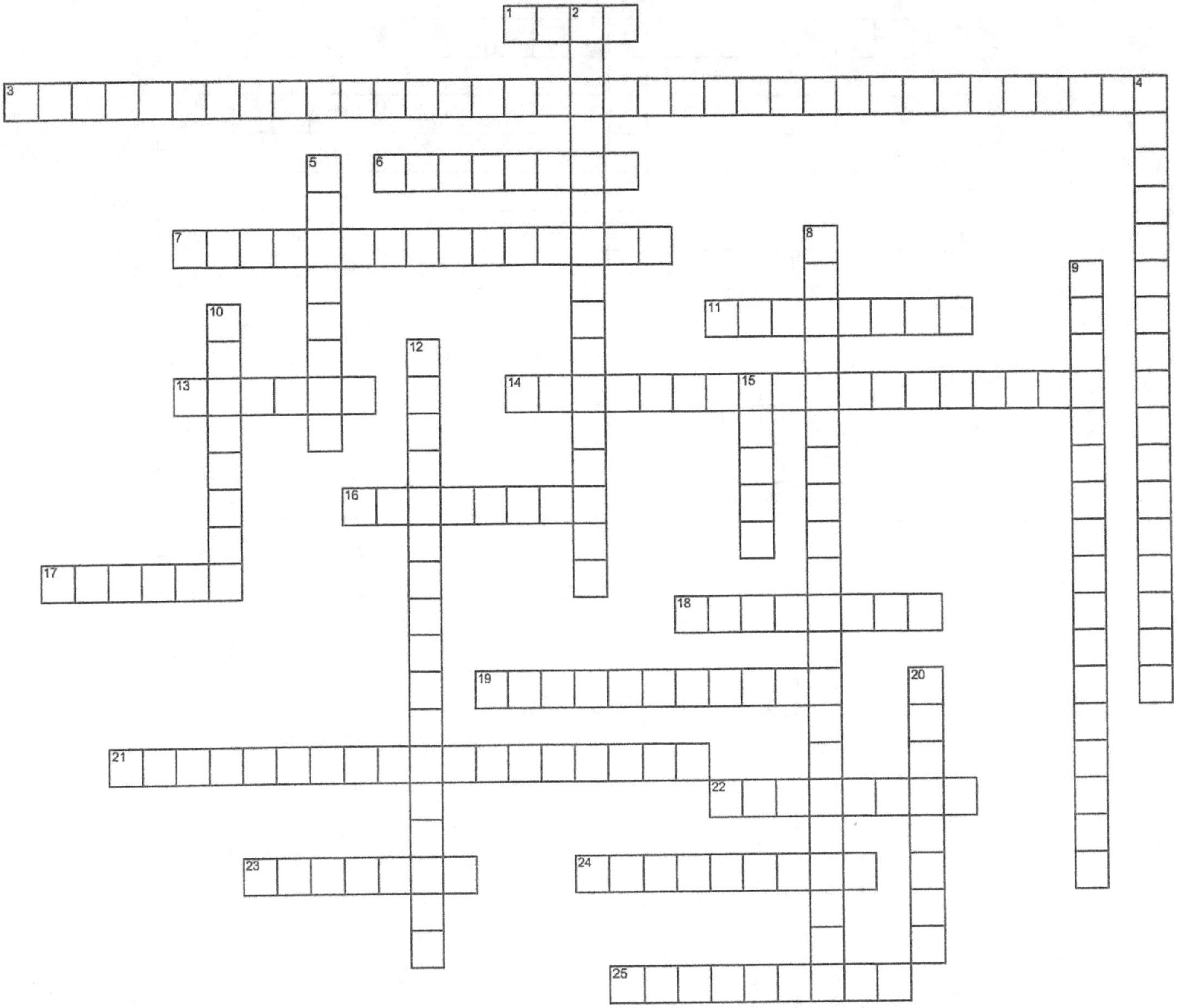

ACROSS

1 Any event or process that can result (directly or indirectly) in economic loss of damage to a facility and/or its reputation
3 H.A.T.C.H. An integrated approach to cultural change (5 wds)
6 United States laws which are passed by federal and state legislatures
7 H.B.V. (3 wds)
11 One who has died
13 Physical harm, pain, suffering, loss of income or reputation
14 Using the best medical practices from multiple disciplines (2 wds)
16 When employees can choose the hours they work, as long as they put in the expected number of hours per time period (2 wds)
17 "tab"
18 A set of records that list each monetary transaction in a facility (2 wds)
19 Lesser governing bodies, such as county commissions, have these instead of statutes
21 F.U.O. (3 wds)
22 Blood vessels that carry the blood from the heart to cells
23 Foreign material. When it enters the body, the immune system mobilizes for an attack
24 There are as many of these as there are employees in a facility
25 Difficulty swallowing

DOWN

2 Limits infiltration of heat, smoke, and fire gases (2 wds)
4 The economic term for the unusual or infrequent (2 wds)
5 Expensive hospital cases
8 This is required for potential residents who may have mental illness or mental retardation, who may require higher intensity and/or frequency of services, or specialized rehab services (2 wds)
9 When noncompliance with one or more requirements can cause serious injury, harm or death to a resident (2 wds)
10 A legally binding agreement between two or more people
12 Confining a resident against his or her will, within fixed boundaries (2 wds)
15 Illegally taking another person's property
20 Interventions to Reduce Acute Care Transfers to hospitals. A quality indicator program that focuses on the management of acute changes in resident's condition in a SNF.

PUZZLE # 3

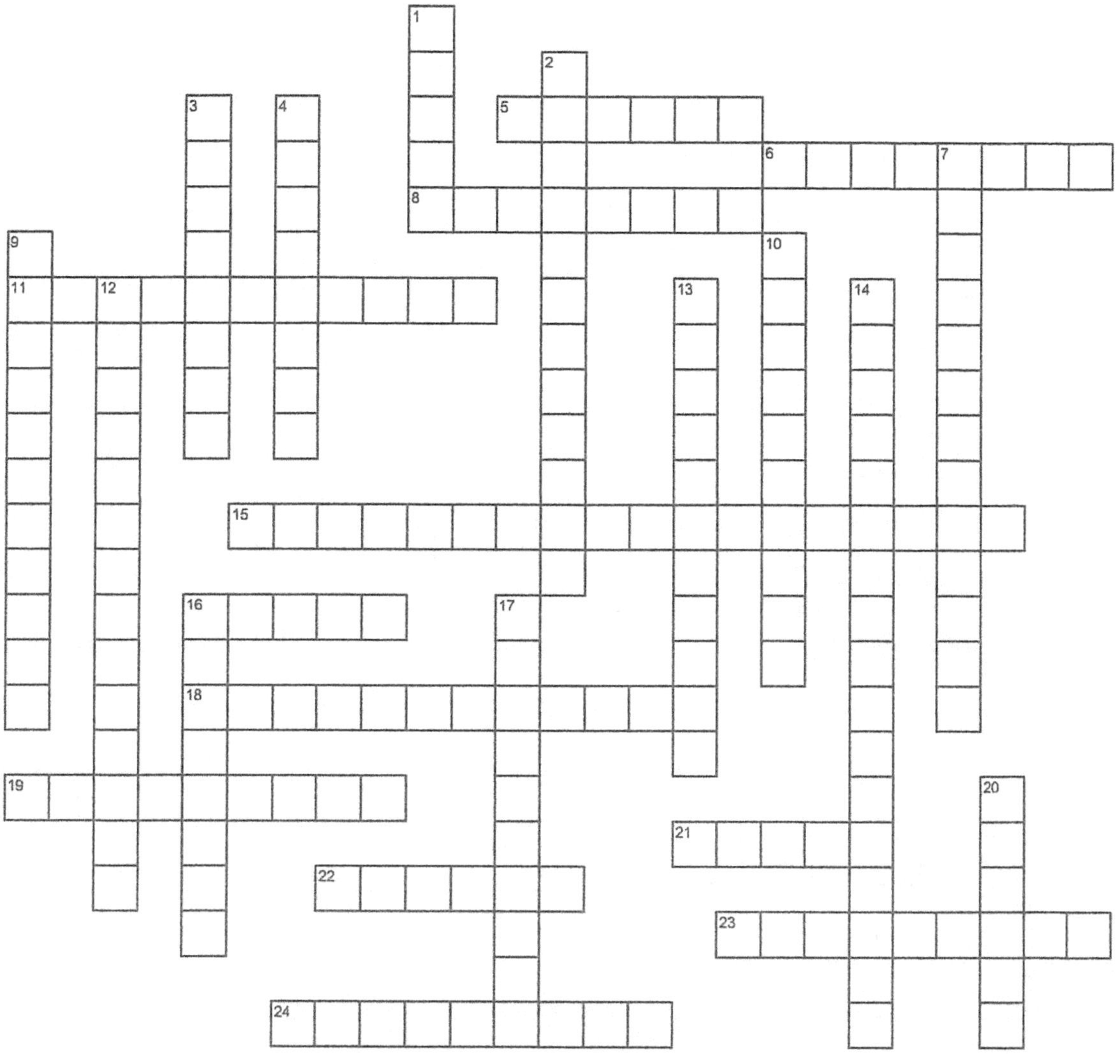

ACROSS

5 A legal term that describes when one side asks for an action favorable to that side
6 Stimulates urination
8 The part of a SNF or NF that is certified
11 Another term for a handwritten will
15 Ice packs, heating pads, baths, massage, physical therapy, and TENS are examples of these. (2 wds)
16 The assessment that occurs in the most recent four months (46-165 days) preceding the target assessment
18 Non-deliberate or premeditated murder, with malice of forethought. (2 wds)
19 An asset that is recognized as a current expense in regular periods throughout the life of the asset. A loan with scheduled, periodic payments of both principle and interest.
21 When is land a depreciable asset?
22 The combining of two companies
23 Charges for supplies and/or services that are not included in the per diem rate
24 Used to reduce pain

DOWN

1 Medicare that covers medication expenses (2 wds)
2 Type of cost that the Administrator has influence over (example: payroll)
3 A party of a lawsuit (either plaintiff or defendant)
4 Policies and procedures must be reviewed how often?
7 The outcome of one's actions
9 A doctor of physical medicine, including body movements and conditioning. May be related to sports medicine
10 Chief accountant of a firm (also called a Comptroller)
12 Used for inventory costing, this method makes the value of goods in inventory lower than that of the goods used to provide services (in the event of inflation) (LIFO) (4 wds)
13 Deliberate, premeditated murder with malice (2 wds)
14 D.O.N. (3 wds)
16 Term used to describe the responsibilities/ duties performed by one staff member
17 A type of quality measure or quality indicator that provides a description of a resident or patient at a specific point in time
20 The personal property that is owned and left at death

PUZZLE # 4

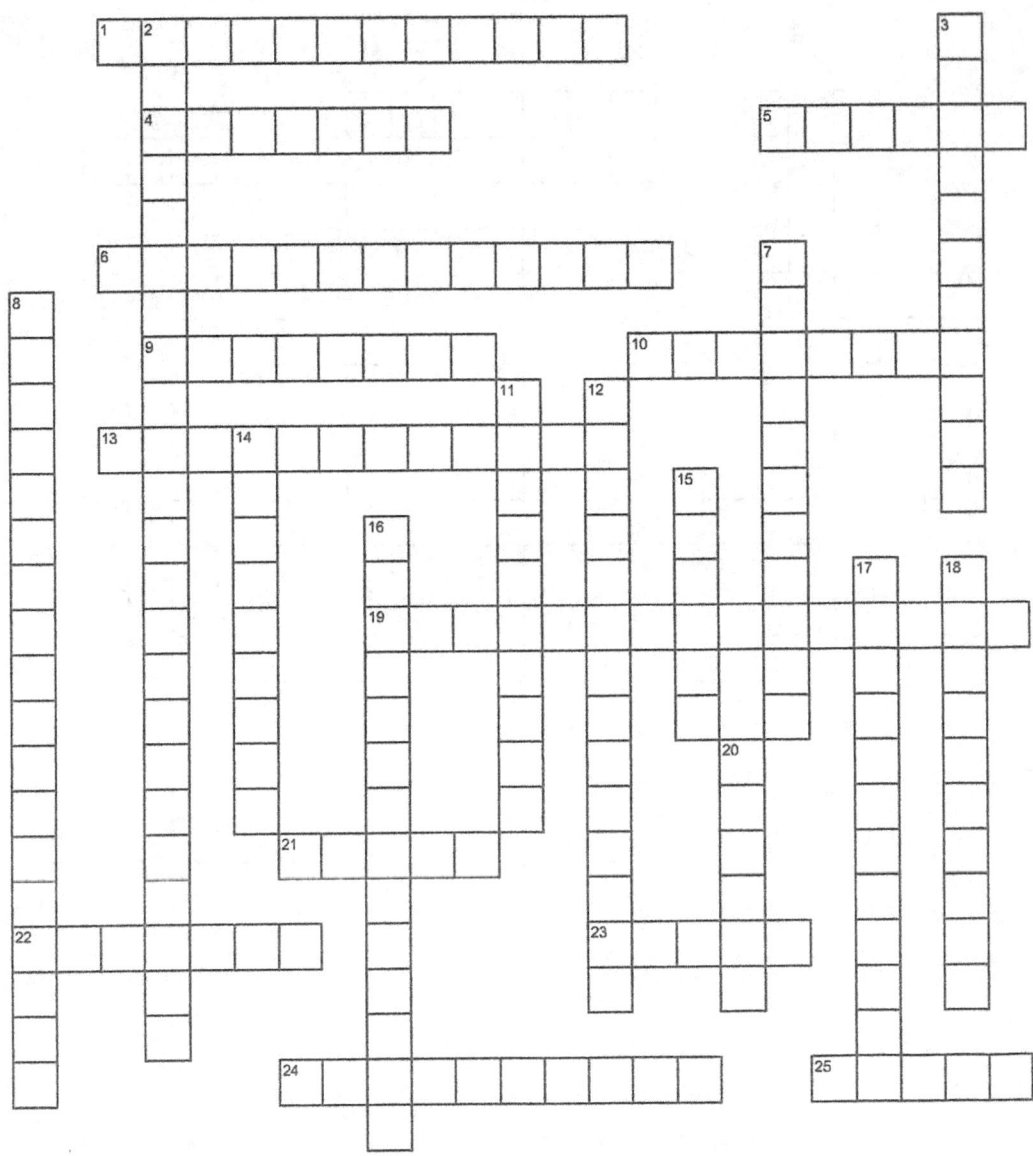

1
2
3
4
5
6
7
8
9
10
11
12
13
14
15
16
17
18
19
20
21
22
23
24
25

ACROSS

1 Term that means "friend of the court" (2 wds)

4 ________ Old Age Security Act. 1930, by F.D. Roosevelt. Provided cash income to those in need, excluded those in public and private institutions, and emphasized short-term acute care. (2 wds)

5 Doors must open _____ means of egress

6 The theory that behavior depends on reward. When reward follows performance, performance improves. The outcome reinforces employee response, positively or negatively.

9 A private party files a lawsuit and becomes the plaintiff. A losing defendant is not incarcerated, but must reimburse plaintiff for losses.

10 The maximum allowed emergency alarm level is 120 ______.

13 A doctor who specializes in the large intestine, rectum and anus

19 Medications that are covered by an insurance company (2 wds)

21 The Administrator is the _____ of the facility

22 Supplemental health insurance sold by private insurance companies (under Federal guidelines) to fill in gaps in Medicare coverage. Assists with days 21-100 of a patient's stay in a SNF.

23 This is used to make someone do something that he or she would not otherwise do. It is a complex concept.

24 Those who express interest in a defined market offer

25 A ph value of ___ is neutral. Less than this is considered acidic, and more is considered basic.

DOWN

2 Enters a risk contract with a state Medicaid agency to provide a specific package of benefits to Medicaid enrollees in exchange for a monthly capitation payment on behalf of each enrollee. (3 wds)

3 A contract between two people to pool their resources and efforts in order to conduct a business operation

7 Litigation is filed by the government, also known as the prosecution. Guilty party may be incarcerated, fined, or executed.

8 Using a protected category as a basis for treating people unequally. When a person or group is singled out and treated less favorably than others. (2 wds)

11 This document lists the specific treatment to be given to a patient. Patient's wishes. (2 wds)

12 S.O.T. (3 wds)

14 The presence of numerous professions in a Nursing Home tend to _______ the Administrators power

15 A problem with red blood cells, that results in the body not getting enough oxygen

16 A promissory note with a five to six year term (3 wds)

17 The current value of a future payment or stream of payments. This estimates fair market value of a potential investment, and is also known as discounted cash flow method (2 wds)

18 A transformational process when nutrients undergo various chemical reactions. The body breaks down the food eaten into a usable form for cells.

20 The unlawful killing of another person. Homicide, with malice of forethought and premeditated intent.

PUZZLE # 5

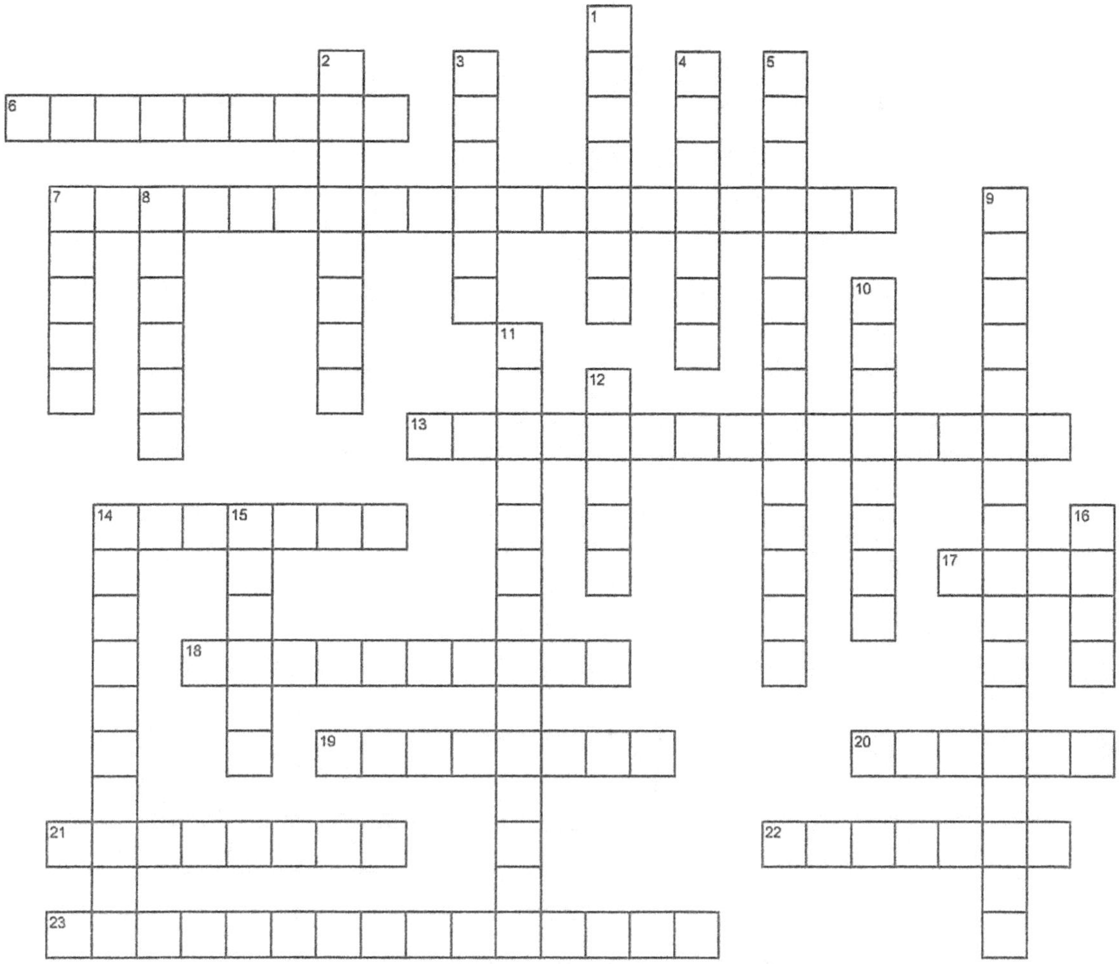

ACROSS

6 Between 1993 and 2005, occupancy rates in SNF's/ NF's _______.
7 A.D.R. (3 wds)
13 N.F. (2 wds)
14 A document issued by the state establishing a corporate entity
17 Standardized pattern of required behavior. The characteristic and expected social behavior of a person
18 A legal procedure, when a defendents property is seized by a court order, pending the outcome of the claim.
19 Smoke and fire alarm systems must be ______
20 Smoke detectors must be no more than ___ feet apart from one another
21 Type of equity that describes fair, appropriate compensation within a facility
22 An amendment to a will
23 A highly detailed plan of specific actions that each employee is expected to follow. (Example: What to do when the fire alarm goes off) (3 wds)

DOWN

1 Smoke detectors must be no more than ___ feet from any wall.
2 The amount of long term debt a facility has in relation to its equity
3 Elements that the Administrator can change, and use to his or her advantage
4 As a quality measure, this assures that all organizational arrangements believed needed are in place, and that services meet consumer needs.
5 The award of a small sum of money, to recognize the invasion of a legal right of the plaintiff (when there is no injury or pecuniary loss) (2 wds)
7 The person who acts on behalf of, and under control of another
8 The answer to what the facility seeks to become
9 Who is responsible for telling residents about any communicable diseases in the facility? (3 wds)
10 The process of identifying, collecting and analyzing information about the external environment
11 A culture within a facility, where resident preferences and past patterns form the basis of decision-making about some, but not all routines. (2 wds)
12 This day leaves a lasting impression. It is the best time for an official welcome, introduction to staff, and tour of the facility
14 The ability to make a will
15 The three most common types of cancer for males are lung, colon, and _______.
16 Between 2008-2012, ______ new facilities opened in the United States, due to the market.

PUZZLE # 6

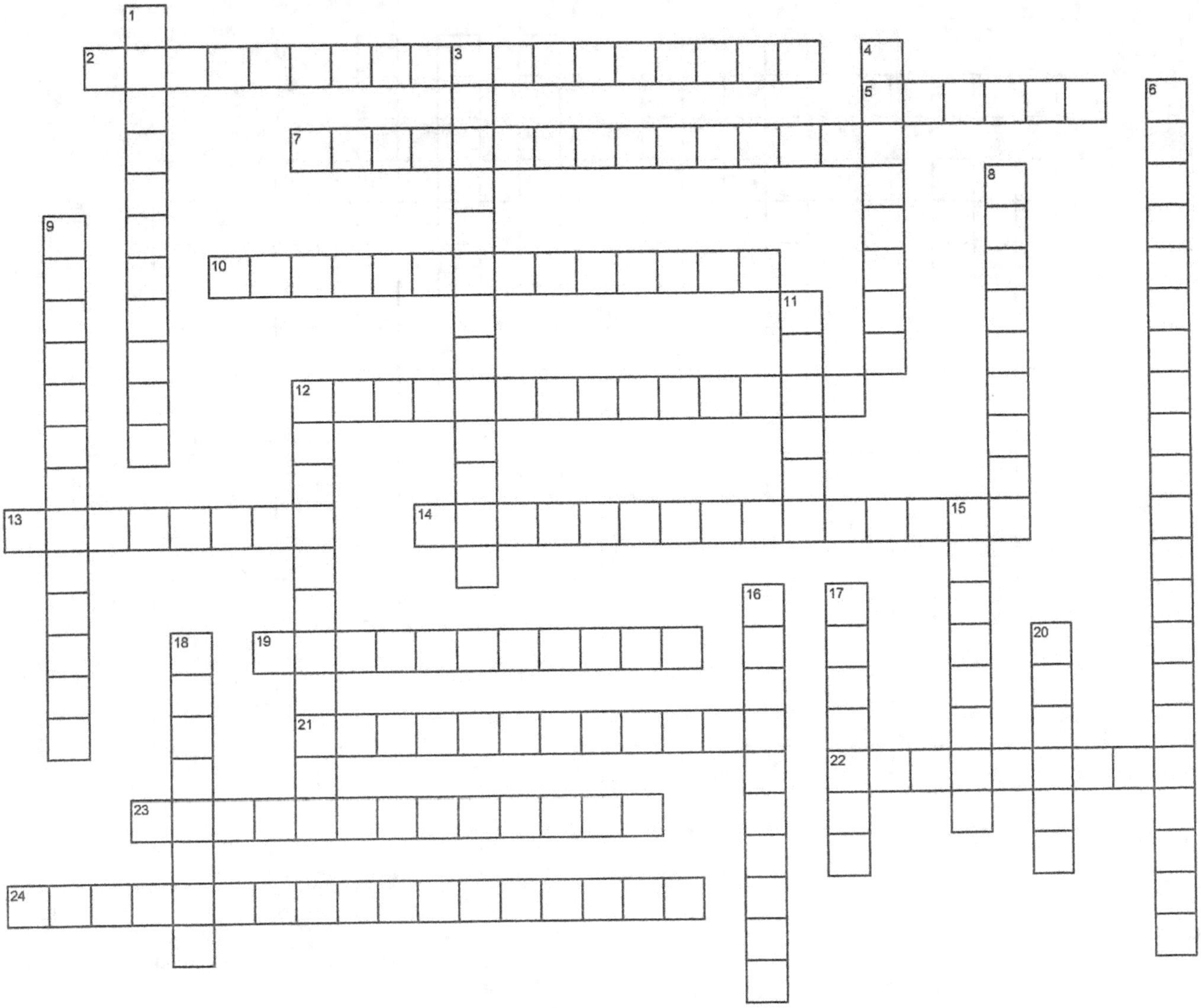
1
2
3
4
5
6
7
8
9
10
11
12
13
14
15
16
17
18
19
20
21
22
23
24

ACROSS

2 The process of deciding which of the applicants best fits a job (2 wds)

5 An accounting concept, where the nursing facility is considered as a whole, but separate from affairs of its owners, managers and other employees

7 The table used by the Centers for Medicare and Medicaid to define severity and scope of federal deficiencies, and to indicate whether plans of correction and remedies are necessary. (2 wds)

10 Considered more safe than a nasogastric tube, because there is less chance of aspiration (2 wds)

12 A culture within a facility, where residents make decisions regarding their routines, and staff organizes their hours and assignments to meet the needs of the residents (2 wds)

13 A term to describe intentional misleading or deception (2 wds)

14 Conduct that is treated as irresponsible, without actual proof. when the act is in direct violation of a safety statute (or is deemed clearly harmful to others) (3 wds)

19 In long-term care facilities, this is driving attention to quality

21 Activities of daily living that are necessary to maintain ones immediate environment, such as cooking, housework, or paying bills.

22 Education offered throughout the work career of the employee, often of a mandatory nature.

23 Excluded from gross income, this allows employees to choose from a selection of two or more benefits consisting of cash or qualified benefit plans (such as medical insurance, life insurance, or sick leave) (2 wds)

24 When a facility is certified for both Medicare and Medicaid (2 wds)

DOWN

1 Doctor who specializes in the brain, nervous system and spinal cord

3 In 2002, the Act that states that publicly held companies must implement internal controls over financial reporting, operations and assets to evaluate strengths and weaknesses of these controls in official documents filed with the Securities and Exchange Commission, and to make regular disclosures regarding the viability of these controls and potential fraud or losses that may affect a company's financial position. (For for-profit facilities) (2 wds)

4 A facility may manage a resident's personal funds if that resident is insured by _______.

6 The study of drug use patterns in a facility (3 wds)

8 A step-by-step, specific method to carry out one policy or task.

9 This determines the skills, knowledge and attitude needed for a specific job (2 wds)

11 Certified Nursing Aids (CNA's) must acquire _____ inservice hours per year

12 A doctor who examines body tissues under laboratory conditions

15 "spec"

16 in 1946, this act funded the building of hundreds of hospitals, long-term care facilities, and other facilities in the United States. (2 wds)

17 Paul ________ founded the first specific remedy in the 20th century. (Salversan, for Syphilis, in 1907)

18 The granting of an alternative requirement in place of a federal or state regulation

20 The granting of a variance

PUZZLE # 7

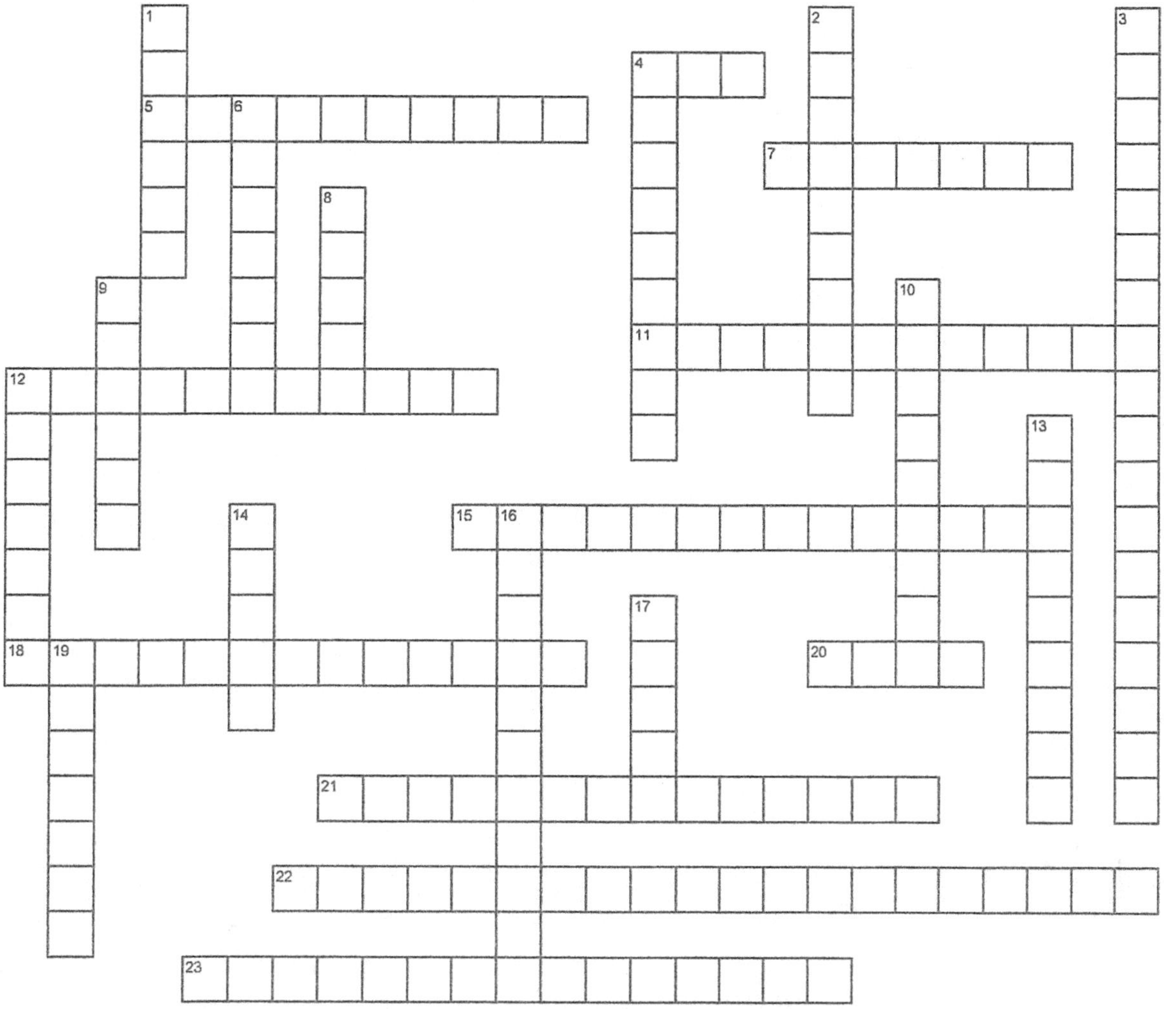

ACROSS

4 Baths and/or showers must be given to each resident _____ times a week
5 this consultant must visit the facility monthly, and must report irregularities to the attending physician or D.O.N.
7 This makes use of accounting information to make decisions regarding how to raise additional funds and how to use given resources
11 O.L. (hours; very costly) (2 wds)
12 When two companies combine, but both keep their separate identities
15 Identifying and solving problems before they get out of hand (2 wds)
18 This area offers the most room for innovation (2 wds)
20 Type of contract where services are provided as needed for non-routine activities (example: a contract for electrical work in a facility)
21 Disease in which the heart muscle suffers from a lack of oxygen due to blockages in the arteries that usually supply that oxygen (2 wds)
22 When a patient's information is overheard by someone else, unavoidably. (2 wds)
23 In England in 1722, this Law stated that the aged, chronically ill, and disabled could live in workhouses, establishing the basis for LTC. (2 wds)

DOWN

1 Money, people, and materials
2 A written statement, under oath, under an officer who has authority to administer oaths
3 Disease with increased resistance in blood vessels in the extremities; disease with obstruction of large arteries in the lower extremities (2 wds)
4 The set point for quality indicators, where the likelihood of a problem is sufficient enough to warrant investigation.
6 The absence of bacteria, viruses, and other microorganisms
8 Illegally taking another person's, or organization's property
9 To set free
10 Employees normally do not outperform their ______. (2 wds)
12 The attempt to inflict bodily harm, or create fear of imminent peril, or the infringement on mental security or tranquility of another. (Does not require actual touching or damage)
13 With oxygen, these permit cells to perform chemical reactions that produce energy
14 In dietary, in case of an emergency, an emergency menu must cover ___ days
16 The type of contractor who performs a certain job and remains in control of the means and methods of performing that job. (Not an employee of a NF; therefore, the NF is not liable for his or her negligence)
17 If a bath or shower is not possible, sponge baths should be given to a resident ______.
19 This type of care is typically for those with six months or less to live, for symptom management, pain relief and support services

PUZZLE # 8

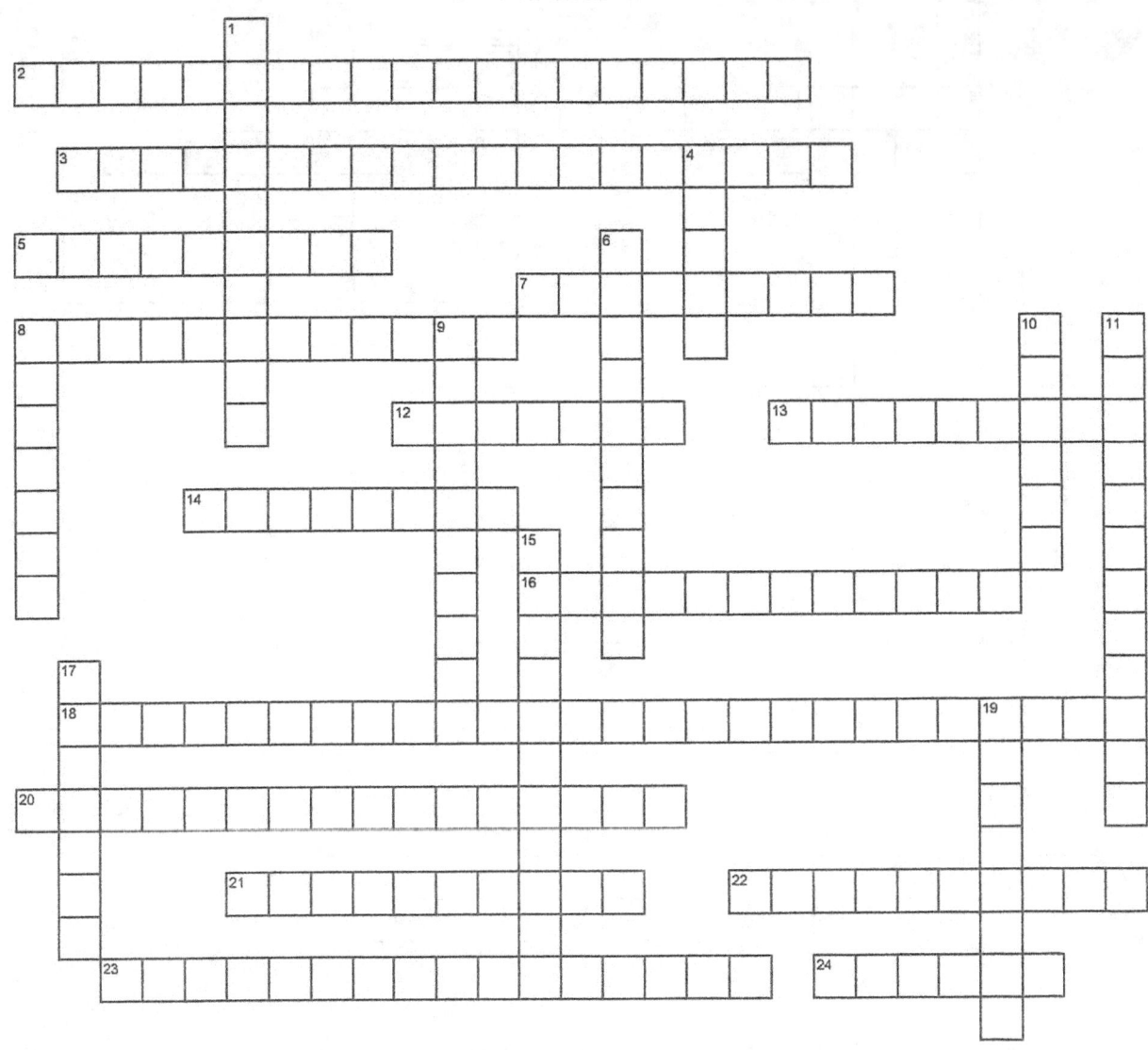

ACROSS

2 These help protect the body. Examples are skin, gastric juices, and urine (3 wds)
3 Money given to an organization to be used in a specific way (aka, Special Purpose Fund) (3 wds)
5 OMN. HOR. (2 wds)
7 Fire extinguishers must be checked ____
8 A decision, process or thing that resolves a conflict. (Example: the final decree in a bankruptcy case)
12 One who computes insurance costs to determine rates to be charged
13 As quality measures, these are related activities that produce a specific service or product (i.e., outcome)
14 Fire extinguishers must be serviced and tagged _____
16 Abnormal illness, condition, or disorder caused by exposure to environmental factors associated with employment
18 E.S.O.P. A benefit plan that gives staff members shares in the facility (4 wds)
20 This hand-held device must be available in every hazardous area, on each floor of a facility. (2wds)
21 One who diagnoses and treats disorders of the foot, ankle, and lower extremity
22 This destroys microorganisms
23 Cognitive readiness, effective readiness, and behavioral readiness (2 wds)
24 This carries red blood cells

DOWN

1 A ___ is appropriate for the task of hiring an Administrator (2 wds)
4 There must be no more than ___ feet travel distance to a Class B or C hand-held fire extinguisher
6 When an organization is unable to pay its debts, it files for this... (This was rare for NF's and SNF's before 2000)
8 This type of drawing is prepared by the contractor, and shows on-site changes to the original construction documents. It shows renovations and/or new construction (2 wds)
9 Doctor who researches, identifies and treats tumors (i.e., cancer)
10 This gives an organization direction, and helps supply enthusiasm
11 The condition of no longer being used or useful.
15 Predicts what the future WILL look like
17 This type of insurance will pay a portion of intermediate care needs at home, with doctor orders from a follow-up to illness or injury. It does not cover custodial or intermediate care in a NF.
19 Preliminary financial statements, based on budgeted amounts, which are developed at the end of the budget process. (2 wds)

PUZZLE # 9

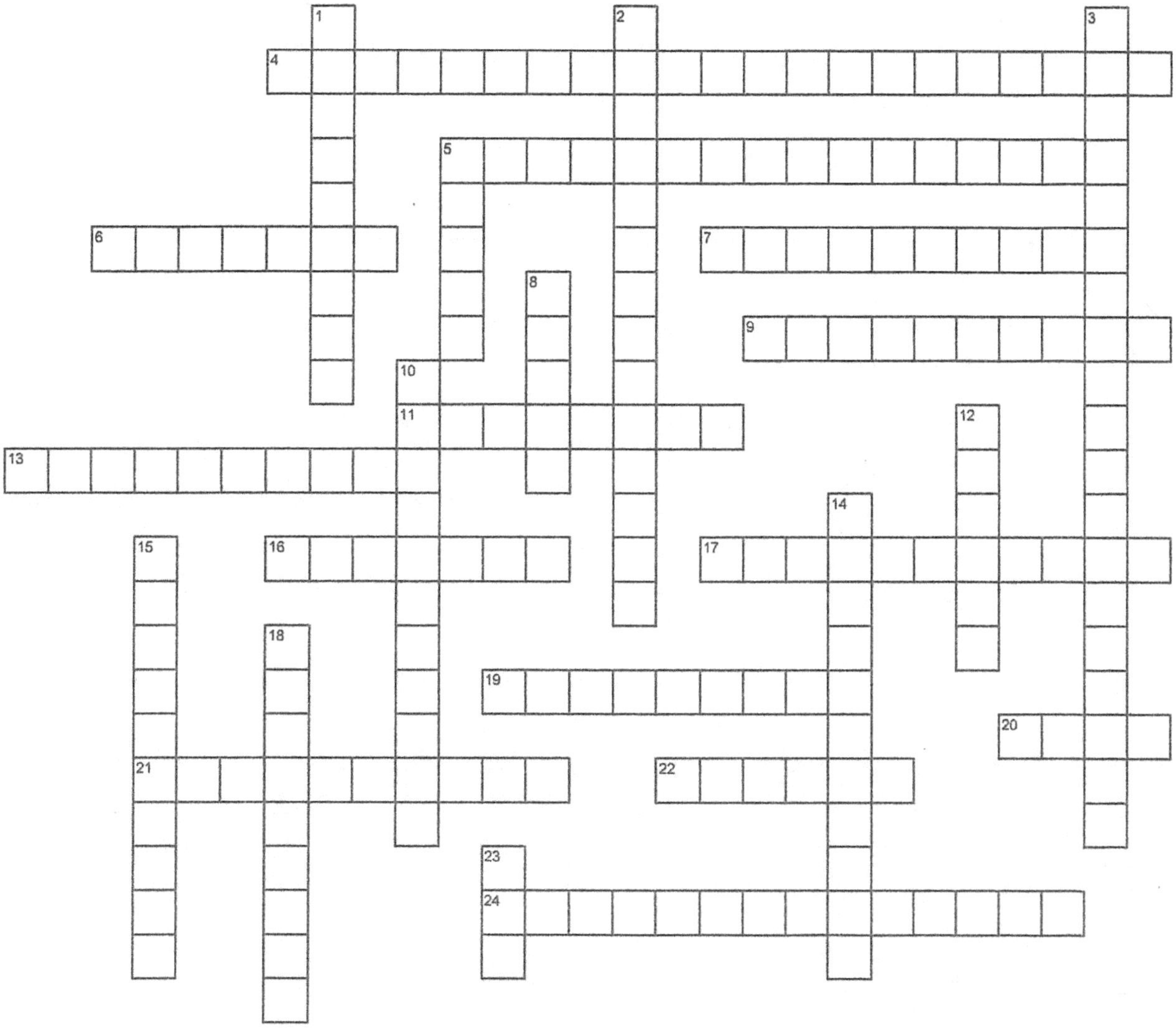
1
2
3
4
5
6
7
8
9
10
11
12
13
14
15
16
17
18
19
20
21
22
23
24

ACROSS

4 A growth strategy, where a company buys a competitor at the same level of services (2 wds)

5 Those who have consumed offered services (in this case, those who are admitted as residents) (2 wds)

6 The most frequent cause of fires in NF's or SNF's is _____.

7 Classifying an expense as an asset because it benefits the facility for more than one year. This enables a facility to recognize the cost of a large investment over a longer period of time (years), rather than only at the time of expenditure.

9 The distance between any room to an outside exit must be no more than ____ feet. (250 feet if an automated sprinkler system is installed) (2 wds)

11 C.A.T.'s have _____ guidelines to follow.

13 If a patient requests access to his or her record, the facility must grant that access within ___ hours (2 wds)

16 "By practice" (2 wds)

17 Hearing loss is most detrimental to, and causes difficulty with ____.

19 How long a job or activity must wait until facilities are available (example: how long it takes to get a room ready for a new resident)

20 Desired type of budget, since income/ expenses vary from time to time

21 Cost = _____. (How well a company uses its assets)

22 All who have an actual or potential interest in using a facility's services

24 This summarizes all payroll checks which were distributed during a pay period (2 wds)

DOWN

1 Derived from past judicial decisions; principles that evolved and expanded from decisions from past trials (2 wds)

2 L.C.D. (3 wds)

3 This determines when results of a course of action are enough to justify the cost of its undertaking (3 wds)

5 Type of stock used by young, public companies that are not listed on any stock exchange. They are sold at a lower price than other stocks

8 According to Life Safety Code, the width of any corridor must be ___ feet

10 V.O. (2 wds)

12 Intentional wrong-doing, without just cause or excuse, with the intent to do harm or inflict injury

14 An offense punishable by less than one year and/or a fine

15 This slows down bacteria growth, but does not kill it. (Example: Hydrogen Peroxide)

18 Type of market that eliminates those who are interested in a market offer, but unable to pay. Eliminates issues related to funds, access, etc)

23 Registered Pharmacist

PUZZLE # 10

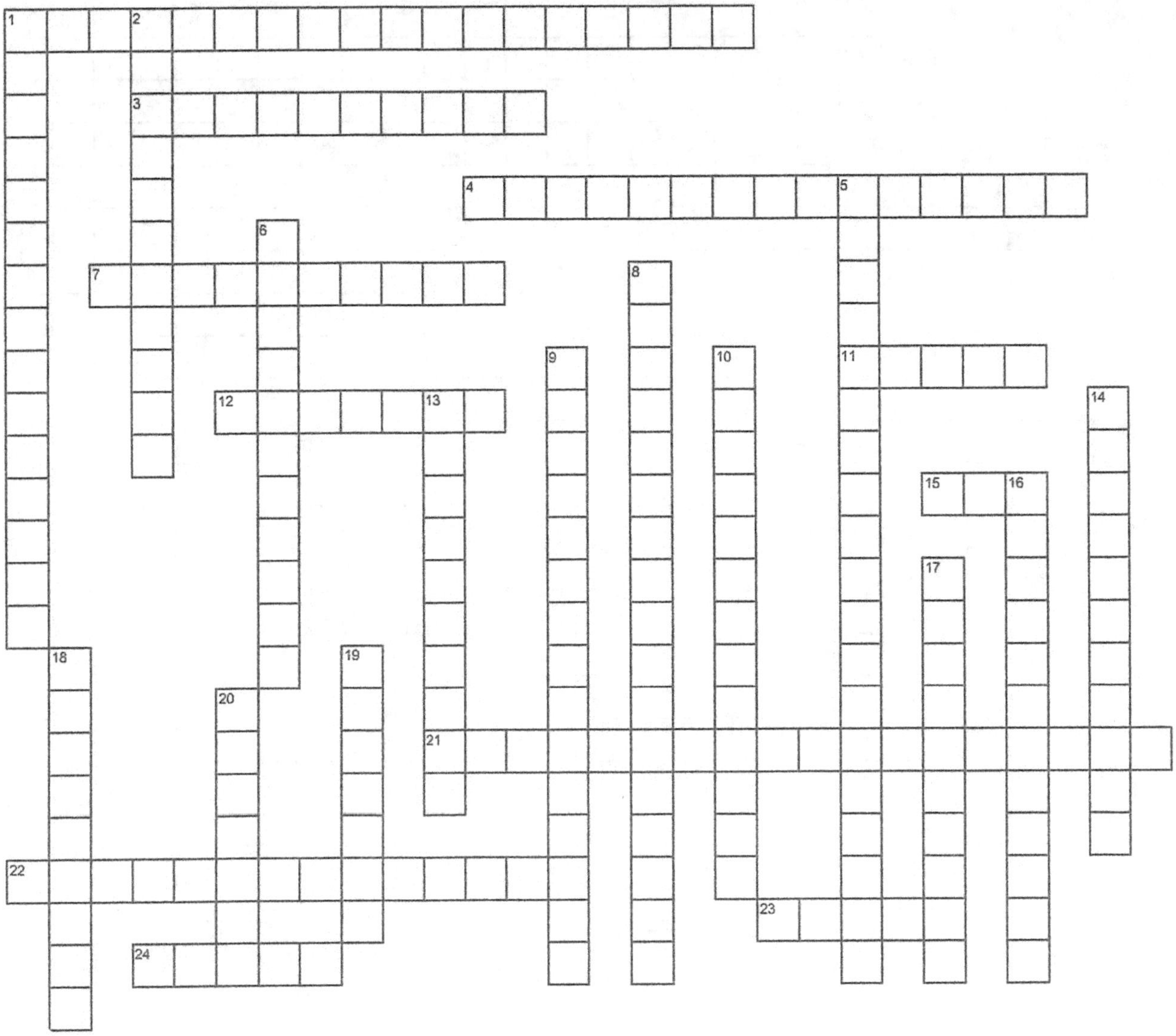

ACROSS

1 Recklessness or carelessness that results in injury and/or death punishable by law. A reckless disregard for another's safety or rights. (To recover damages, the plaintiff would have to prove duty to care, breach of duty, injury and causation) (2 wds)

3 This compensates a resident (or the state acting on his or her behalf) for any loss of resident funds that the facility holds and manages (due to incompetence, negligence, or dishonesty) (2 wds)

4 C.A.T. (3 wds)

7 A non-invasive, drug-free medical practice which places emphasis on the interrelationship of musculoskeletal and other body systems. Focuses on total body health by treating and/or strengthening musculoskeletal framework.

11 Medical orders must be reviewed every ___ days by the attending physician, nurse practitioner or physician assistant.

12 This type of diet helps rebuild tissue (2 wds)

15 If a patient requests a written copy of his or her medical record, the facility must provide a copy within ___ days. The facility may charge a fee for each copy.

21 A control tool that shows the relationship among activities that make up a project. (3 wds)

22 Type of impact in quality and/or staffing that increases revenue and/or decreases operational costs.

23 Carefully developed ___ help compare what happens to what was predicted

24 This carries white blood cells

DOWN

1 A standardized, mandatory statistical collection method; A list of names and numbers of all accounts used by a business (including accounts in assets, liabilities, owners equity, revenues and expenses) (3 wds)

2 A type of negligence, where a person improperly performs an act, resulting in injury to another. (Example: wrong-side surgery)

5 This employee must have a Bachelor's degree, 1000-hour dietetic internship, and pass the national exam. He or she must also acquire 15 continued education credits per year. He or she may be full-time, part-time or a consultant. (2 wds)

6 This principle states that a business must use the same accounting method from one period to the next (i.e., year after year). If the method is changed, it must be disclosed in the notes of the financial statement.

8 What is subtracted from gross pay to arrive at net pay? (2 wds)

9 The present value of an investment in excess of initial amount invested (3 wds)

10 This helps prevent clotting

13 When one is summoned and goes to court

14 Federal requirements promulgated to "flesh out" the statutory requirements in the Social Security Act

16 Type of acute, chronic illness caused by inhalation, absorption, ingestion or direct contact to an environmental factor at place of employment

17 Verbal orders for medications may be given to a licensed nurse, physician, or ____.

18 Judging if the actual results of a facility's efforts achieve the outcome proposed in the plans.

19 The percentage of falls of those age 65 and over which account for deaths

20 Amount per patient, per day. Daily allowance for expenses. Used to compare rates to other facilities, and to monitor cost of services provided. (2 wds)

PUZZLE # 11

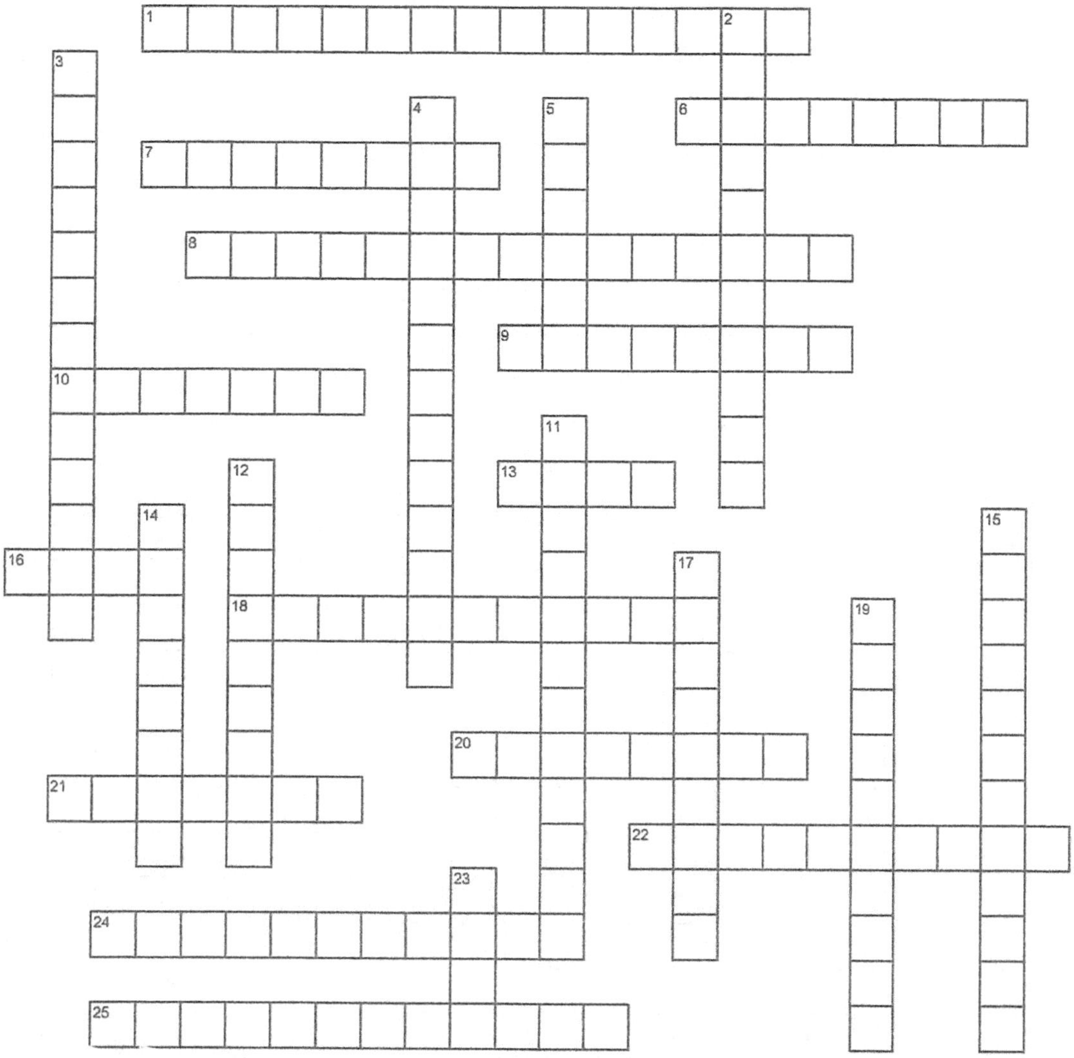

ACROSS

1 Doctor of the ductless gland system, to include the pituitary, thyroid, pancreas, and adrenal glands.

6 The three parts of a Resident Assessment Instrument are the MDS, CAT's, and the ____ (2 wds).

7 Type of equity that describes what staff at other facilities are earning

8 An item or right with no physical substance, that provides economic benefit. An example is "reputation". (2 wds)

9 A focal, creative, psychic event where knowledge, thought, feeling and imagination are fused into action

10 "surg"

13 Approximately how many facilities were chain-owned between 1993-2005?

16 The number of days a facility has to inform a state survey/ certification agency about any incident involving mistreatment, neglect or abuse

18 Giving employees space to innovate, listening to and acting on resident suggestions, and leading by walking around are all examples... (2 wds)

20 Predicts what the future should look like

21 A future-looking concept that makes use of past accounting data to make needed decisions

22 The necessary explanation of a companies financial position and operating results. This includes pending lawsuits and other liabilities.

24 There must be no more than ___ feet travel distance to a Class A hand-held fire extinguisher (2 wds)

25 Given by an independent CPA, in order to determine the reasonableness of a facility's financial statement (2 wds).

DOWN

2 The approach to hiring that identifies the most valid predictors of job success, and then uses weights in a formula to choose among applicants for a position

3 This relieves smooth muscle contraction

4 R.O.M.; Helps prevent contractures, benefits those with limited mobility, and helps prevent pressure ulcers (3 wds)

5 In dietary, weekly menus are retained for ____ months.

11 The mistreatment or neglect of those under the care of a health care organization (or home health organization) (2 wds)

12 A judicial decision that may be used as the standard in future cases.

14 Type of power that describes how well employees and residents identify or admire the facility's Administrator. (one of two best types of power an Admin. can have)

15 When nine or more medications are given to a resident (including vitamins).

17 The making of teeth

19 The study of peoples efficiency in their work environment.

23 A claim on property as security for a debt owed. This does not include title or ownership to a property.

PUZZLE # 12

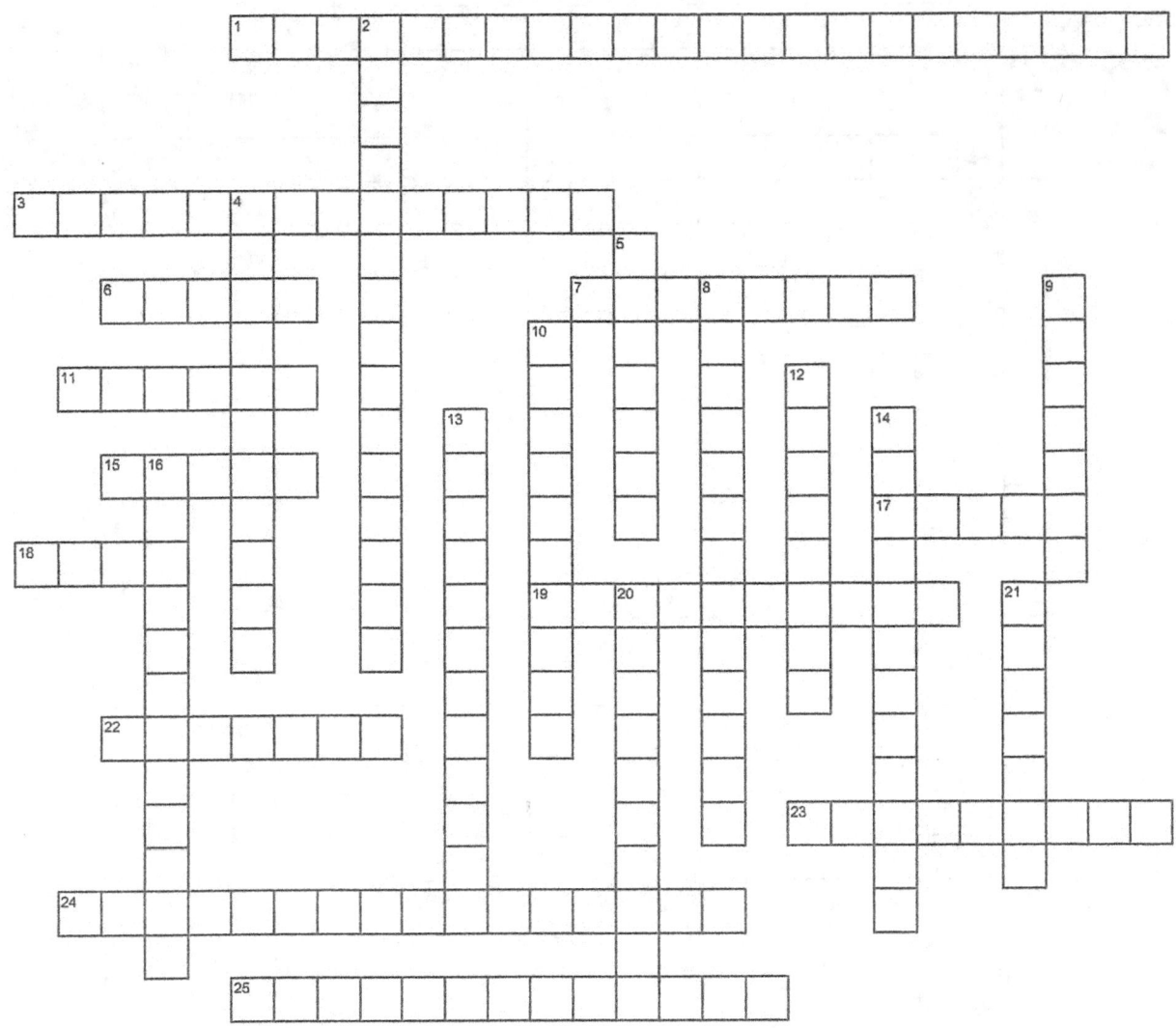

ACROSS

1 C.O.L.A. (4 wds)
3 A way to rank providers based on how they compare to each other on separate quality indicators. The higher a ranking, the more apt the provider is to have a care concern. (2 wds)
6 where the ends of two bones meet
7 Insurance that covers stolen merchandise, furniture, fixtures and equipment
11 The concept of ___ is an organized or complex whole. It is an assembling or combining of things or parts, forming a complex or single whole
15 On an income statement, revenues are listed ____
17 Statements of organizational goals of a facility
18 "u"
19 Fixed costs plus variable costs equal ____ (2 wds)
22 The amount earned from selling products or services
23 An organization's logo. It may be a symbol, a design, or specific coloring/lettering (2 wds)
24 A method to analyze financial statements. This method converts each item on the income statement, balance sheet or other report to a percentage of some total item on the same document. This is useful when compared over time, or compared against another facility. (2 wds)
25 An on-site federal survey, to determine if the provider meets the requirements to participate in the Medicare and/or Medicaid programs (2 wds)

DOWN

2 These vary per unit with the change in volume (3 wds)
4 Type of negligence; a failure to act when there is a duty to act as a reasonably prudent person would. (example: failure to order medical tests)
5 Three dimensions of ____ are structure, process, and outcome
8 Someone who studies old age, and the process of becoming old
9 The work done by an organization; the actual giving of care
10 A judicial order to someone to do or refrain from an act
12 Pressure in the eye, due to increased fluid, when fluid does not drain properly
13 When redness surrounds areas of skin which may become infected
14 A long-term lease for life equipment or property. Expenses are reported as assets and long-term liabilities on the balance sheet. The asset is amortized. (2 wds)
16 An organization that handles claims from nursing facilities, hospitals, and home health agencies
20 One who commits a tort (2 wds)
21 The results of efforts made, and measurable impacts on residents (which determine the quality of services)

PUZZLE # 13

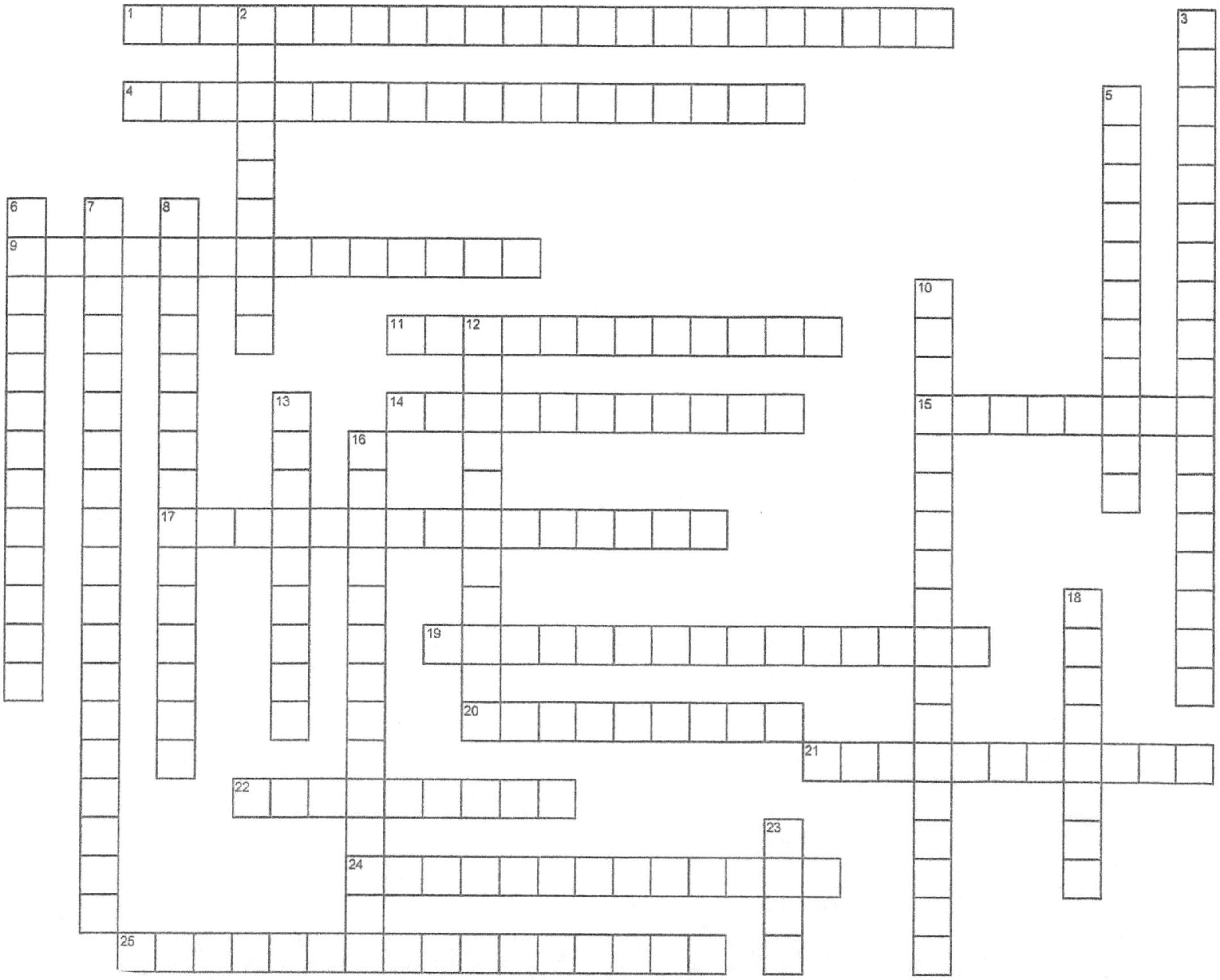

ACROSS

1 Type of multi-state, regional contractor responsible for administering both Medicare Part A and B claims. Under the MMA of 2003, he or she is mandated to process claims. (2 wds)

4 A market so competitive, all participants have no control over price (2 wds)

9 Short-term lease, with a limited number of years.(2 wds)

11 Money that is set aside to meet pension plans (2 wds)

14 The person who receives proceeds or benefits under a policy. Someone who may receive money from a trust, will or life insurance policy

15 to depreciate; to gradually write off the initial cost of an item

17 Its purpose is to help a department achieve its mission and accomplish certain goals and objectives (2 wds)

19 This log contains original entries, and lists all bills sent for services rendered. It is divided by payor type (i.e., private pay, Medicaid, Medicare, etc). (2 wds)

20 When a facility sells some or all of its hard assets to a leasing company for cash, and leases those assets back over time.

21 Negative figures, net losses, are shown in ______ on financial forms

22 Individually identifiable health information, transmitted or maintained in electronic format (or other medium) is called _____.

24 A legal term, meaning one must prove the facts in a dispute. In criminal cases, "reasonable doubt". In civil cases, 51%. (3 wds)

25 These help organize MDS information, and include instructions regarding Resident Assessment Instruments. They used to be called RAP's (Resident Assessment Protocol's). (3 wds)

DOWN

2 An increase in the general price level

3 An expense that costs more than $500.00-2500.00 and has a useful life of more than one year. An item that is intended to be used past the budget period. Also includes money spent to add value or life to fixed assets (2 wds)

5 A term that means upcoding (2 wds)

6 Facility assets used as collateral to secure short-term working capital loans from banks and other lenders (2 wds)

7 Expansion, by moving forward or backward within an industry (2 wds)

8 The reduction in the sales of a product caused by the introduction of another similar product by the same facility or organization

10 These change with volume, or need. (3 wds)

12 Type of infection that develops after a resident is admitted to long-term care

13 Someone who dies without a will

16 A material in its usable form, which will not aid combustion or add appreciable heat to a spreading fire

18 A provision for uncollectable accounts receivable is called an allowance for ____(2 wds)

23 A civil wrong, other than breach of contract. Examples include assault, battery, false imprisonment, and negligence

PUZZLE # 14

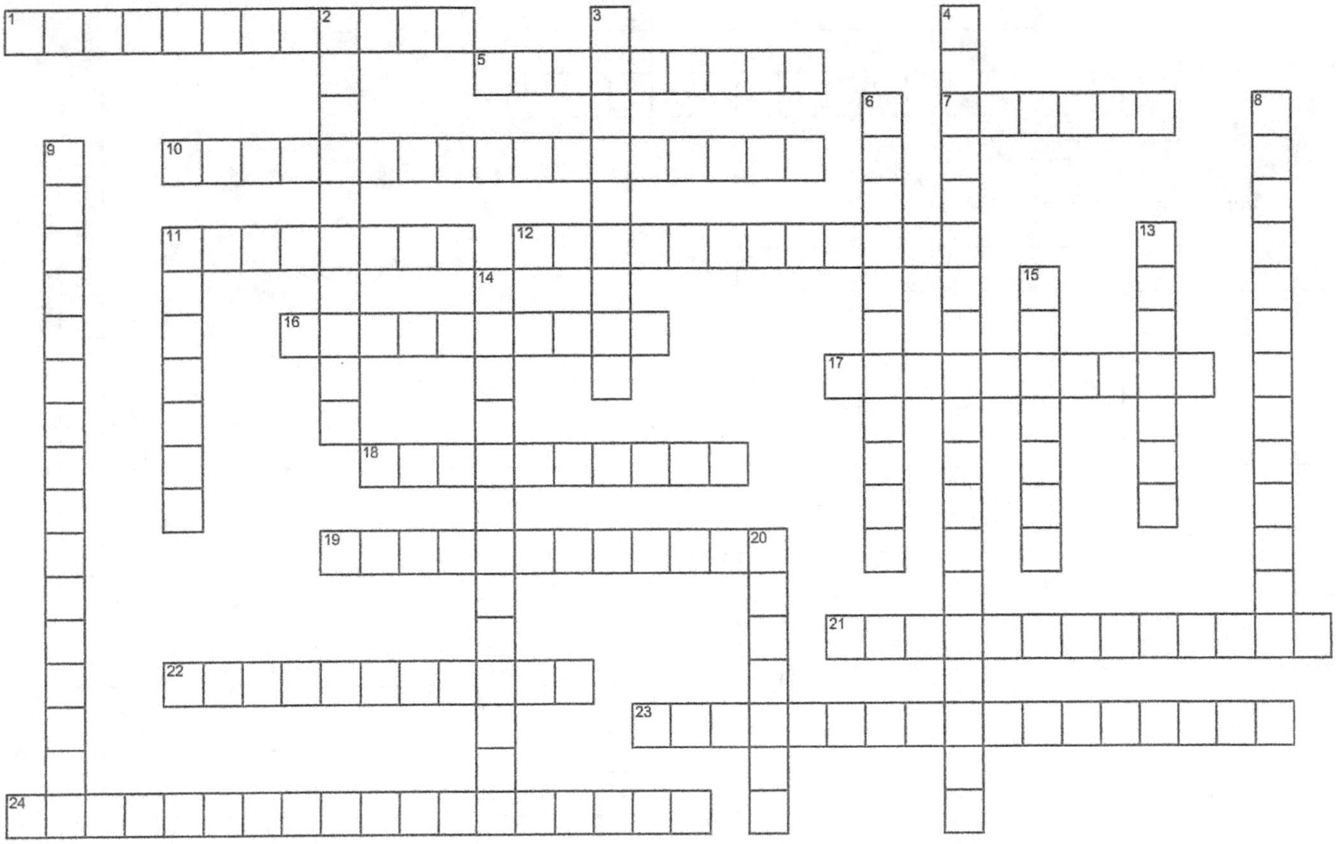
1
2
3
4
5
6
7
8
9
10
11
12
13
14
15
16
17
18
19
20
21
22
23
24

ACROSS

1 When a company buys back a portion of its outstanding stock (2 wds)

5 The three most important financial reports for stakeholders are the balance sheet, the income statement, and the statement of ____. (2 wds)

7 Shellfish I.D. tags must be kept on file for ____ days

10 The assets of a company available to common shareholders. What each share is worth, based on historical stockholders' equity costs maintained in a company's accounting books. (4 wds)

11 The three federal government branches are legislative, executive and _____.

12 Type of drug that affects the brain. Used to change, modify or alter a person's behavior or mood.

16 A disease with no cure, which causes tremors, rigidity, muscle stiffness and bradykinesia

17 Type of care for terminal residents. Alleviates suffering even when there is no cure

18 Type of theory in which the level of motivation to perform is a mathematical function of the expectation people have about future incomes, multiplied by the value the employee places on these outcomes

19 The review of a job description, and the activities essential for doing that job. (Step two of establishing training needs) (2 wds)

21 A doctor who specializes in the treatment of lungs

22 Another term for resident care costs. (2 wds)

23 Type of program devised by CMS in 2002, to serve consumers and providers by providing access to quality measures, assistance and resources of state-organized quality improvement organizations. It compiles information about residents on eight situations or conditions called quality measures, and makes that information available to consumers (2 wds)

24 A "clean option"; a report that meets all GAAP (Generally Accepted Accounting Principles) requirements (2 wds)

DOWN

2 In 1974, this Act gave federal staff the right to examine their human resource records, including letters of reference, unless they waived their right when they requested the letter (2 wds)

3 Percentage of those in the workforce, who were union members in 1947

4 Step four of the accounting cycle (final step) (2 wds)

6 An association of shareholders created by law and treated by the law as "a person". An artificial person with a legal existence entirely separate from those who compose it.

8 The use of government powers to keep prices either up or down. (2 wds)

9 An auditor's report of the facility financial statement, that points to a particular limitation (2 wds)

11 Step one of the accounting cycle

13 Type of leadership, where the focus is on serving others

14 An action significantly difficult or expensive, when considered in light of factors (such as an organization's size or resources) (2 wds)

15 Oral defamation of character

20 Type of continuous care, given to treat a medical condition. It is ordered by a doctor, and delivered by medical workers 24 hours a day. A treatment plan is devised, and supervised by a physician. It is provided in a certified facility.

PUZZLE # 15

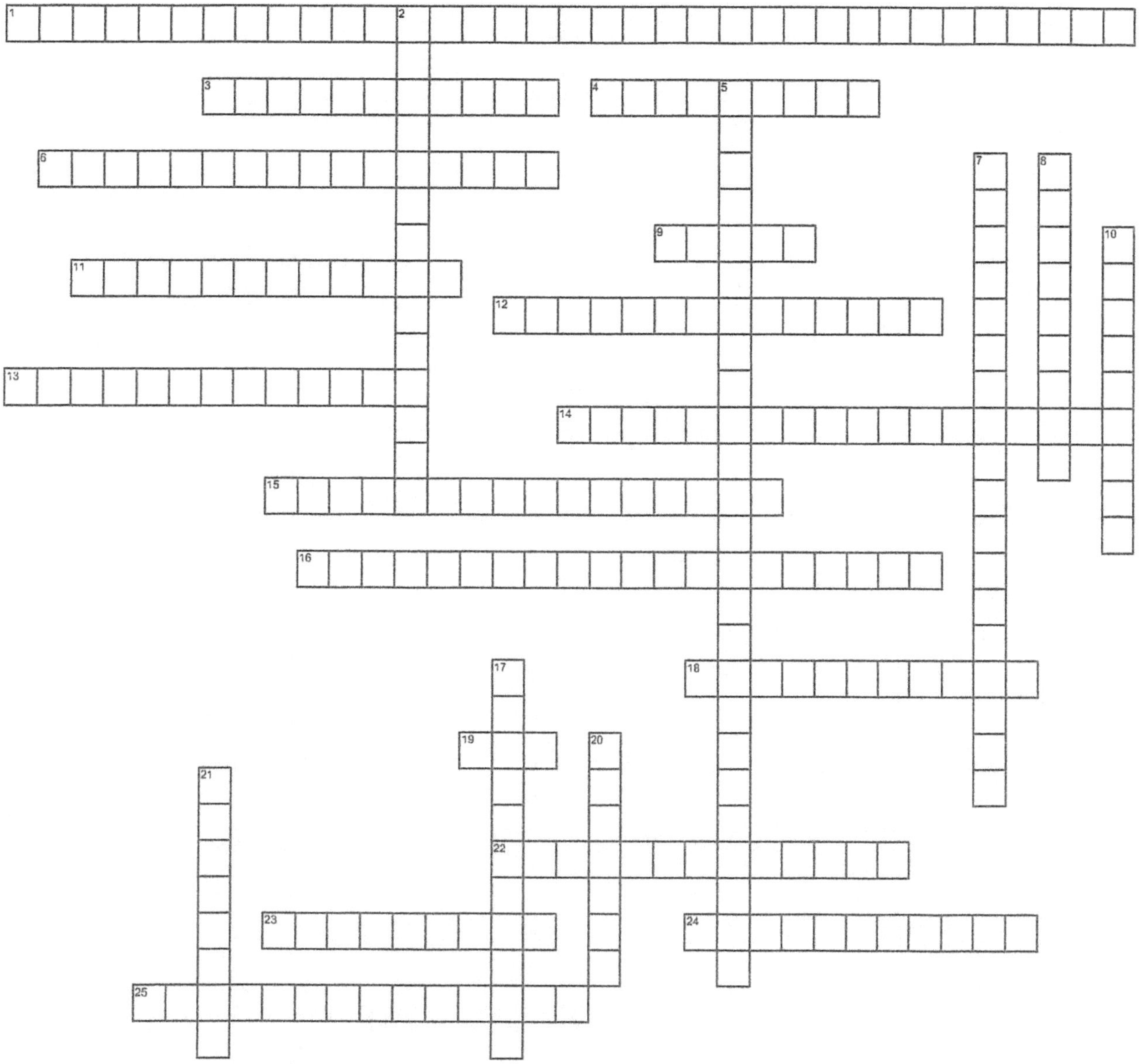

ACROSS

1 A.A.R.P. This organization has over 33 million members age 50+. The organization represents their interests. (4 wds)

3 Interest charges used to measure the market in corporate bonds are reflected in these. (100 of them = 1% point of interest) (2 wds)

4 One element used to establish that negligence has occurred. (There must be a reasonable connection between a defendants negligence and the resulting damages to the plaintiff)

6 This type of leadership is participatory, holistic, and organizationally-driven. Its focus is on educating, supporting and caring for each other

9 Type of legal venture between two companies, where there is a cooperation toward the achievement of common goals

11 Medical condition that causes sharp, burning pain 1-4 hours after eating, nausea, weight loss, and/or bloody stool (2 wds)

12 When someone is distracted with personal issues, an employee may misinterpret a manager's comments as hostile. This is called _____. (2 wds)

13 Department in a facility that generates revenue (usually through resident care). Also, cost centers that focus on costs related to bringing in revenue) (2 wds)

14 Provides education and resources for improving quality of life for elders and for recapturing a meaningful work life for their caregivers (1991) (3 wds)

15 Step two of the accounting cycle (2 wds)

16 Measures to prevent the transmission of infection resulting from contact with blood or other body fluids, or materials with blood on them. These are mandatory, under guidelines from both the United States Public Health Services Centers for Disease Control, and OSHA. (2 wds)

18 When the risk is spread or split among multiple parties

19 Skilled Nursing Facility

22 The rate of return available in the marketplace on investments that are comparable in terms of risk and other things like liquidity. (3 wds)

23 The Uniform Assessment Instrument (UAI) must be completed upon _____.

24 This type of negligence refers to situations where an injury is a result of negligence by both the defendant and the plaintiff. Oftentimes, the plaintiff can recover damages, despite his or her own negligence. (example: Slippery shoes, slippery floor)

25 Particular capabilities of a company that separates it from others and serves as a basis for growth or diversification into new lines of business (2 wds)

DOWN

2 Step three of the accounting cycle (2 wds)

5 The first federation of labor unions in the United States, in 1886. Formed by skilled workers. (4 wds)

7 Income - expenses = profit. Another term for this profit is _____. (3 wds)

8 The term coined to suggest giving employees a proprietary sense of participation in the facility and its goals through treating employees as members of a team

10 A party whose legal rights have been invaded, or who has suffered a loss or injury

17 Any funds for restricted use are recorded here. This is a record of assets donated to an organization, that are restricted by donors or outside parties to certain, specific uses, and are separated and categorized as such. (2 wds)

20 Percentage of those in the workforce, who were union members in 1990

21 The Uniformed Service Employment and Reemployment Rights Act (USERRA) of 1994 protects those in the _____.

PUZZLE # 16

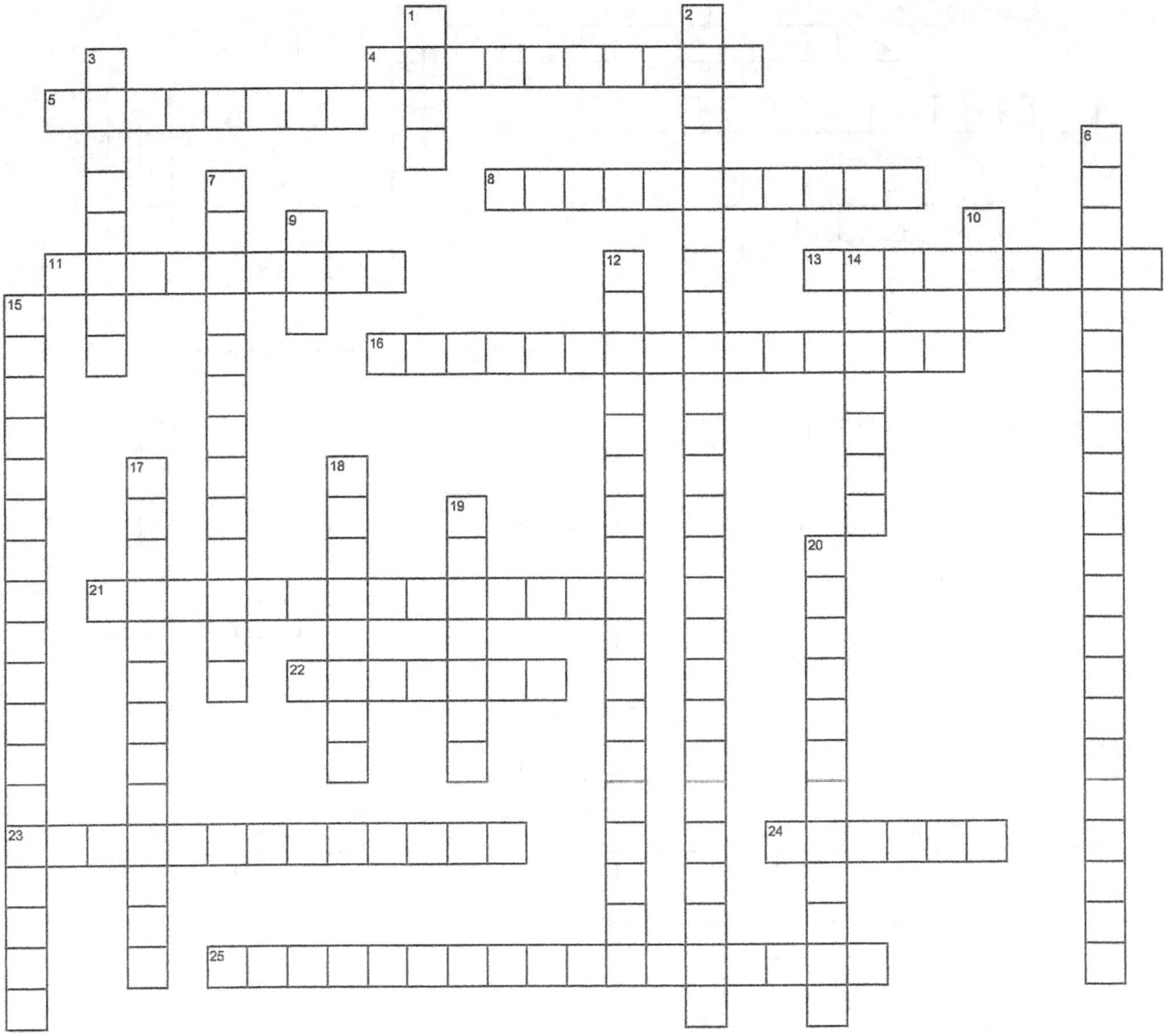

ACROSS

4 Type of communication among peers
5 Type of power, where the employee believes that the Administrator has the ability or inclination to punish bad behavior (with warnings, firing the employee, requiring a resident to leave, etc) (Also known as punishment power)
8 Type of accounting where each transaction is recorded twice. The sum of debits equals the sum of credits (2 wds)
11 These must be no more than 34-38" from the floor.
13 Triple net leases, where the lessor's role is only that of the financier. Lessor assumes no liability regarding the operation of the facility (3 wds)
16 Events that arise out of damage or injury that took place during a policy's term. (The insurance company pays for claims for events occurring during the term or policy, regardless of when claims are filed) (2 wds)
21 The cost of acquiring an asset that is depreciated over several time periods. (2 wds)
22 This may be interpreted with many variations by surveyors. It is a term to describe recognizing resident individuality
23 Shares of common stock issued to the general public, but repurchased by the issuing company (2 wds)
24 This mineral acts as a buffer. It dissolves substances in the blood stream, and monitors the amount of body fluid.
25 D.R.R. This reviews the drugs being taken by a resident to determine their effects. (3 wds)

DOWN

1 The legal term for a compilation of statutes and regulations
2 This tracks 1700 stocks in 91 industries (4 wds)
3 Type of communication used by a supervisor to his or her staff. (Examples: department meetings, in-services, bulletin boards, mail)
6 Where appeals from trial judgments are held. Each state has at least one. (2 wds)
7 These are used as fuel for the body. Two sources are sugars and starches.
9 Number of cups of fluid per day, which must be offered to a resident
10 The lessee is responsible for the maintenance of property, taxes, and insurance with this type of lease
12 The amount by which sales exceed variable costs (such as supplies, labor) of a service. The resulting, left over money may go toward fixed costs. (2 wds)
14 Earnings Before Interest, Taxes, Depreciation, and Amortization and Rent. This is used to analyze operating profitability before non-operating expenses. However, this is not used as a measure of cash flow.
15 R.O.I. Measures the earning power of a facility's assets. (3 wds)
17 The legal term to describe the person who transfers the property of one who dies without a will to those who succeed in ownership
18 Type of damages used to punish a defendant and deter future bad conduct (also called exemplary damages)
19 This mineral builds bones and teeth. Also helps clot blood.
20 This staff member must have a Bachelors degree, one year of experience, and must be full-time if the facility has 120+ beds (2 wds)

PUZZLE # 17

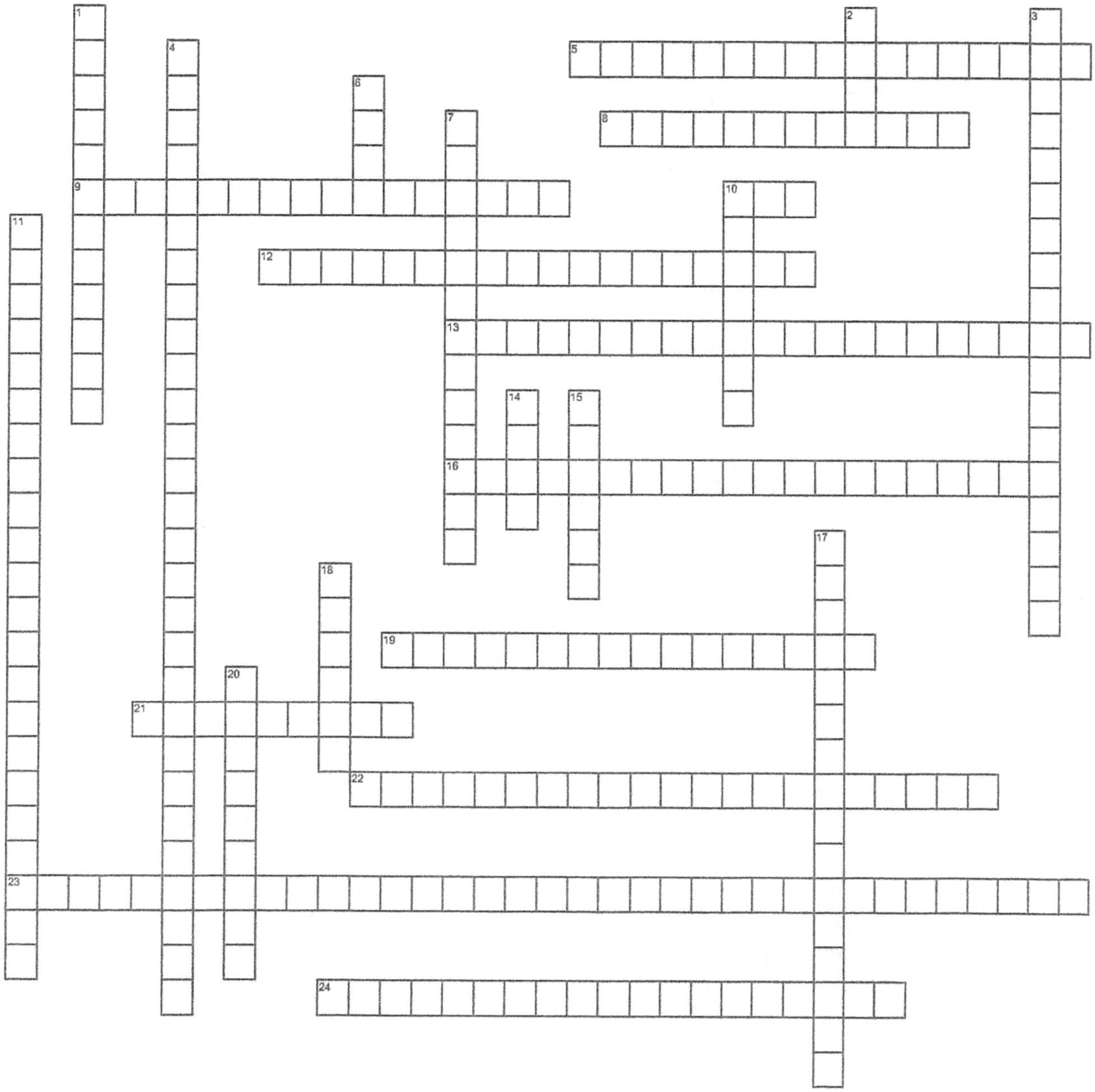

ACROSS

5 When a facility must match the revenues earned with the expenses incurred, to generate the revenue during the period covered by a report (2 wds)
8 The ___ of nursing homes will be obsolete in ten years (2 wds)
9 When a drug is given without a medical reason (2 wds)
10 Centers for Medicaid and Medicare Services (abbreviation)
12 An evaluation of the intent and actions of a competitor (2 wds)
13 A system for antibiotic review and control (2 wds)
16 Significant conditions or events that exist for only one to three cases (3 wds)
19 E.D.K. (Some states require a permit for this) (3 wds)
21 This mineral aids with muscle contraction, and is contained in fluids and tissues
22 Determines the optimum amount of materials needed to be ordered on a regular basis. (Cost of possession versus cost of acquisition) (3 wds)
23 Devoted to medication error prevention and safe medication use (5 wds)
24 Influencing employee behavior through reinforcement (2 wds)

DOWN

1 Qualified potential residents that the facility makes an effort to attract (2 wds)
2 This mineral builds healthy red blood cells that can carry oxygen
3 Type of staffing when someone can be on-call twenty four hours a day, seven days a week. More likely to be utilized in larger facilities with a lot of Medicaid patients (3 wds)
4 M.I.S. The study of how an organization communicates and processes information to maximize effectiveness of management and to further the organization's objectives. A computerized system that assists with information collection, storage and retrieval methods that assist in work processes. (3 wds)
6 Since 1990, the most active union seeking to organize nursing home workers (abbreviation)
7 The increase or decrease in total costs that results from the output of one more or one less unit (example: one more bed, one more nurse?) (also known as incremental costs) (2 wds)
10 A facility or product that generates cash (2 wds)
11 This is considered the most effective tool for an Administrator's success (2 wds)
14 Three types of capital market securities are preferred stock, common stock and ___.
15 The elderly have a decreased ability to recognize _____
17 When an insurance company pays for claims made only during the term of a policy, and only for events which occurred during the term of a policy (3 wds)
18 Corporations that are authorized by the federal government. (examples: towns, counties, radio and television stations, the United States Postal Service, Public Broadcasting System)
20 Laxatives or purgatives are considered this

PUZZLE # 18

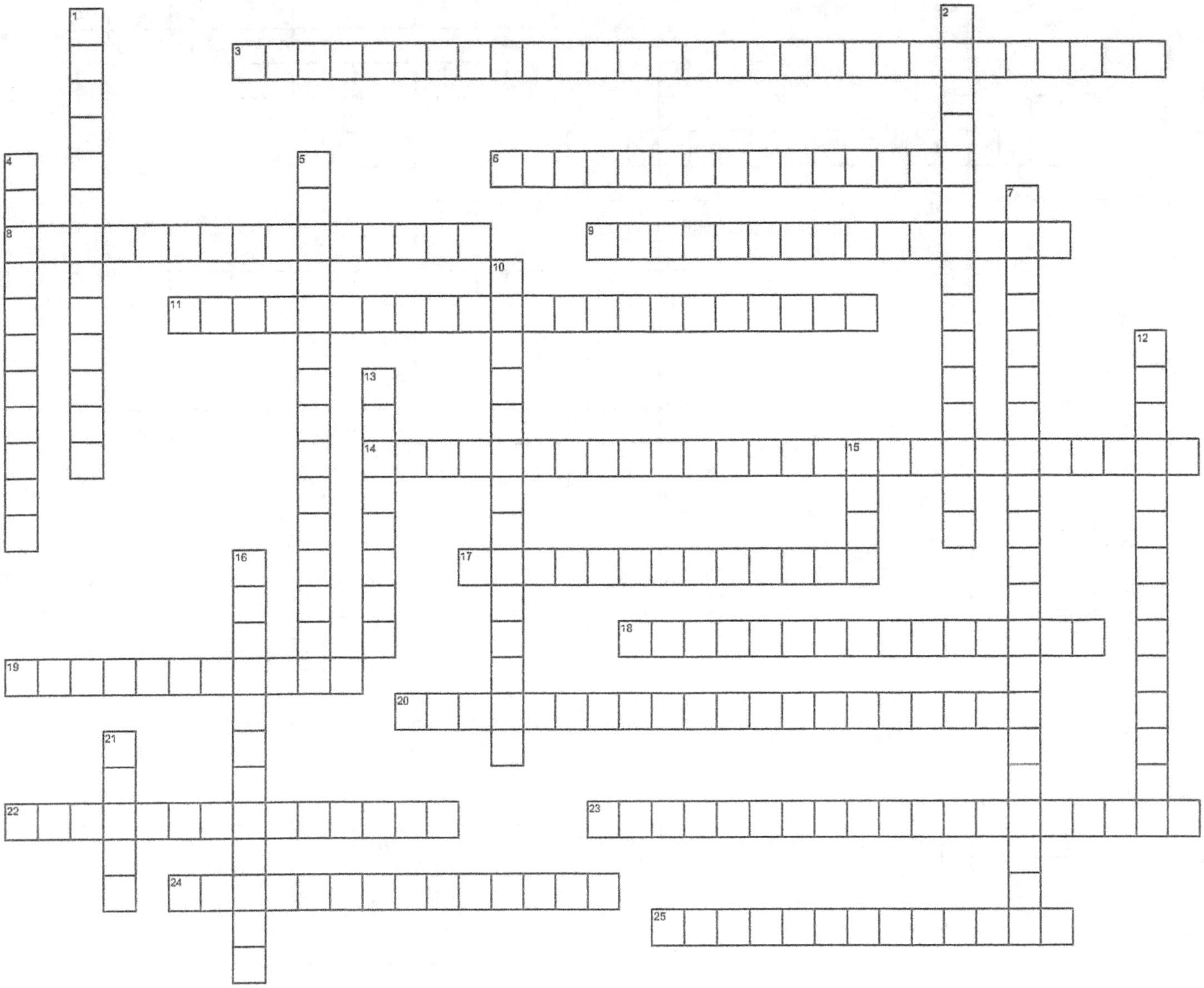

ACROSS

3 H.C.B.S. (5 wds)

6 Any decision or organizational practice that appears impartial but has adverse effects on people in a protected class (example: irrelevant height or weight requirements for a job) (2 wds)

8 Amount of square feet per person in an inpatient treatment area (like the therapy room) (3 wds)

9 This type of care promotes independence, helps maintain muscle strength and prevent falls, and prevents contractures and pressure sores (2 wds)

11 The exchange of information and the transmission of its meaning. (2 wds)

14 In 1978, this act was an amendment to the Civil Rights Act of 1964, designed to protect pregnant women in the workplace (3 wds)

17 This determines what goes on in a facility and between the facility and the outside community (2 wds)

18 An example is when a pharmacist and nurse discuss side effects of a drug, and the nurse finds the words intimidating (2 wds)

19 Short-term, temporary relief to those who are caring for family members (2 wds)

20 The last valid will by a decedent (4 wds)

22 There are two sources for _____. One is judge-made common law, based on societal values. The other is specific law; legislative law resulting in rules and regulations. (2 wds)

23 L.B.W.A. (4 wds)

24 One advantage of L.B.W.A. is _____. (2 wds)

25 This is done when there is a change in the ownership or administration of a facility (2 wds)

DOWN

1 R.B.C. (3 wds)

2 An unlawful act or deception for personal gain. A result of a lapse in ethics. (3 wds)

4 When a facility is required to increase the proportion of minority (or female) workers (2 wds)

5 This person may serve as the attending physician, but must keep that job apart from his or her other job (2 wds)

7 Weekly checks of equipment, revolving inspections (every 4-6 weeks), upkeep of buildings and equipment, and monthly tests of equipment are all considered _____. (2 wds)

10 N.P.O. (3 wds)

12 Unequal treatment; unequal or adverse impact

13 A person or organization that furnishes equipment or services

15 Every communication is likely to have ___ levels of meaning

16 Doctor who specializes in mental disorders

21 A social harm that is punishable by law

PUZZLE # 19

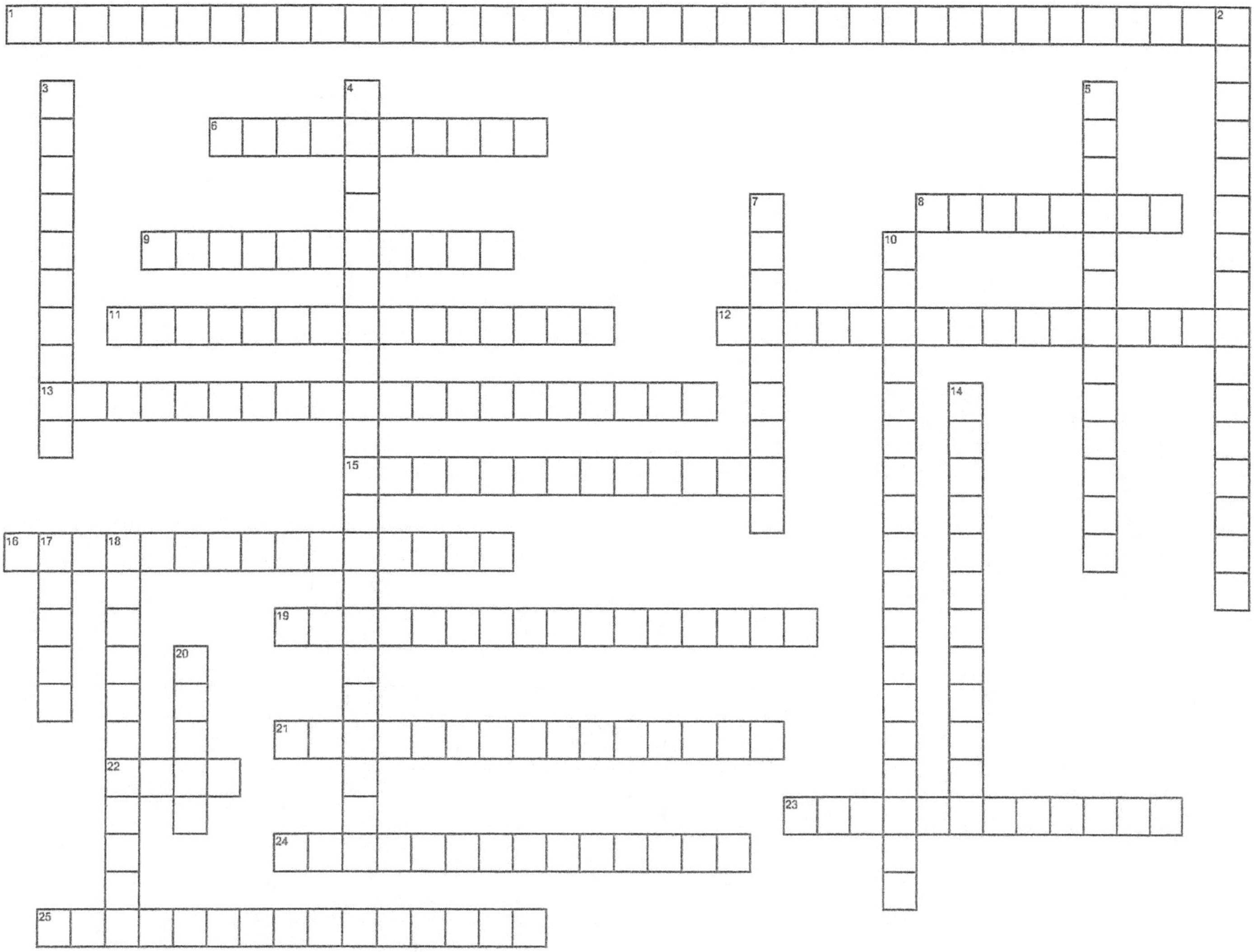

ACROSS

1 G.A.A.P. A set of rules that dictate how books and financial statements are prepared. Consistent standards of accounting. (4 wds)

6 Amount of square feet per person, in a bedroom (2 wds)

8 A written court order to appear in court.

9 A distinct unit within a product line that is different on purpose in some way (2 wds)

11 When an emphasis is on a product's benefit that is valued by an entire market, but is not offered by competition

12 This staff member's credentials vary from state to state, and is also known as a Community Life Coordinator (2 wds)

13 Any refurbishment made to leased property (such as painting, a new roof, etc) (2 wds)

15 To avoid conflict, a manager gives high ratings on everyones evaluations. This is called _____, (2 wds)

16 Term meaning that every organism moves toward death (2 wds)

19 An asset used by a facility to provide services for more than one year, that will not be sold during the course of operations. (2 wds)

21 When two companies combine and one no longer exists (2 wds)

22 True or False: The Medical Director of a NF may be either part-time or full-time

23 This destroys pathogenic organisms

24 A doctor who treats rheumatic and arthritic diseases

25 A contract to receive money at a later date (2 wds)

DOWN

2 If this occurs among employees, an investigation must take place, but no suspension necessarily occurs. If this involves a resident and an employee, however, the employee is suspended while under investigation. (2 wds)

3 Conduct that gives cause for legal action

4 When a facility has minor deficiencies or violations, but the facility generally meets the intent of federal or state requirements (2 wds)

5 When the selection rate of any racial, ethnic, or sex group is less than 80% of the rate of the group with the highest selection rate (2 wds)

7 Pre-trial devices used by lawyers to gather information about the case. Used as a method of facilitating pre-trial settlements and reducing surprises. (examples: depositions, interrogations)

10 This is created by private individuals for non-governmental purposes (2 wds)

14 The restorative therapy program is developed by _____ (2 wds)

17 Borrowing money. The lender and borrower must agree on the purpose for borrowed money.

18 The process of locating prospective staff

20 The requirements for the role of Medical Director are brief and ___.

PUZZLE # 20

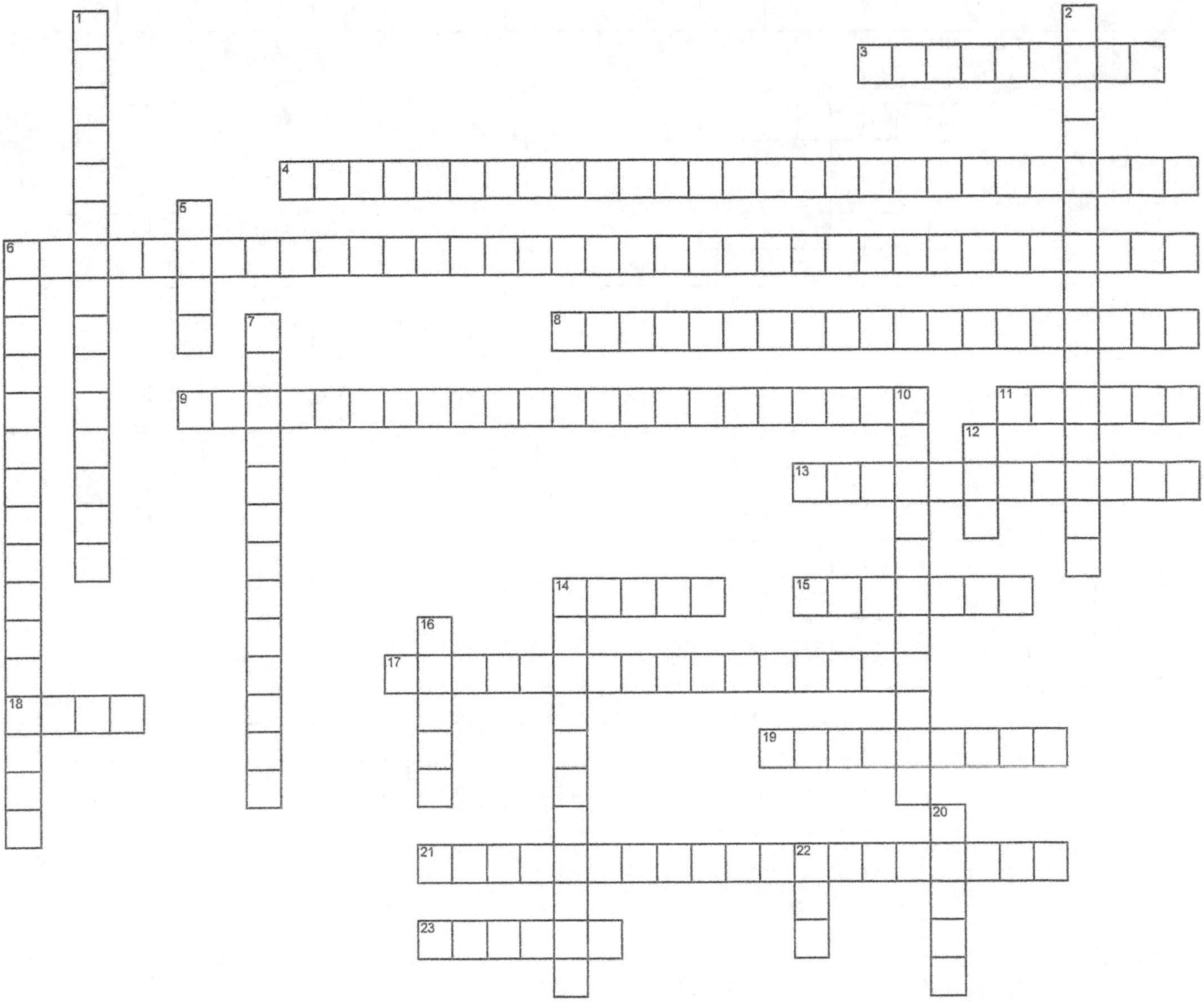

ACROSS

3 This must be between 9-54" off the floor (2 wds)

4 A program that coordinates the delivery of primary, preventive, acute, behavioral and long-term care services. Also, promotes the use of home and community-based behavioral and long-term care services, in Virginia. (3 wds)

6 In 2000, this Act stated that the number of registered nurses, LPN's and CNA's directly responsible for resident care on each shift must be posted in a visible place. (5 wds)

8 Per-day or per-instance fines resulting from deficiencies in the quality of care or resident safety following a CMS survey. (3 wds)

9 This ratio shows the effect that price change has on income. The formula is percentage change in sales divided by change in price. (4 wds)

11 The voluntary relinquishment of a right or privilege. (Regulatory agencies or governments may issue these to exempt companies from certain regulations)

13 The Civil Rights Act of 1991 permitted _____ damage, such as money lost, emotional pain and suffering, and loss of enjoyment of life. It also permitted punitive damages.

14 Which type of Medicare covers outpatient visits, doctor visits and private pay patients who receive therapy? (2 wds)

15 The status of care provided to a resident

17 A term that refers to interpolation. (2 wds)

18 True or false: For non-therapy Medicare Part B services, skilled nursing facilities can submit the bill or have an outside provider bill Medicare directly

19 A doctor who specializes in treating the kidney, bladder, and reproductive organs

21 Stock or bond that can convert into capital stock at a future date. (2 wds)

23 A contract for temporary insurance until a permanent policy can be issued

DOWN

1 Also known as the Autocratic Approach, this is when the Administrator does the budget (3 wds)

2 This constricts blood vessels

5 This explains how real or personal property is to be disposed

6 This group of people assume legal responsibility for establishing and implementing policies in a nursing facility. They develop an organization's mission and goals, strategic plans, programs, policies and procedures, and performance evaluations. All nursing facilities must have one. (3 wds)

7 Costs that fluctuate with changes in volume. When volume and costs rise or fall at the same percentage. (examples: medical supplies, dietary costs) (2 wds)

10 The most organized facilities have no _____ of work

12 For each period of illness, a Medicare patient must pay the equivalent of ___ day of care in a hospital, from day 1-60.

14 In the accounts payable department, purchase orders must be _______.

16 Each Medicare patient has a lifetime reserve of ___ days, which they can use after day 90, if they choose.

20 He said that management should avoid setting too specific objectives that guide an organization over an extended period of time

22 A 200+ bed facility may have ___ mid-level managers

PUZZLE # 21

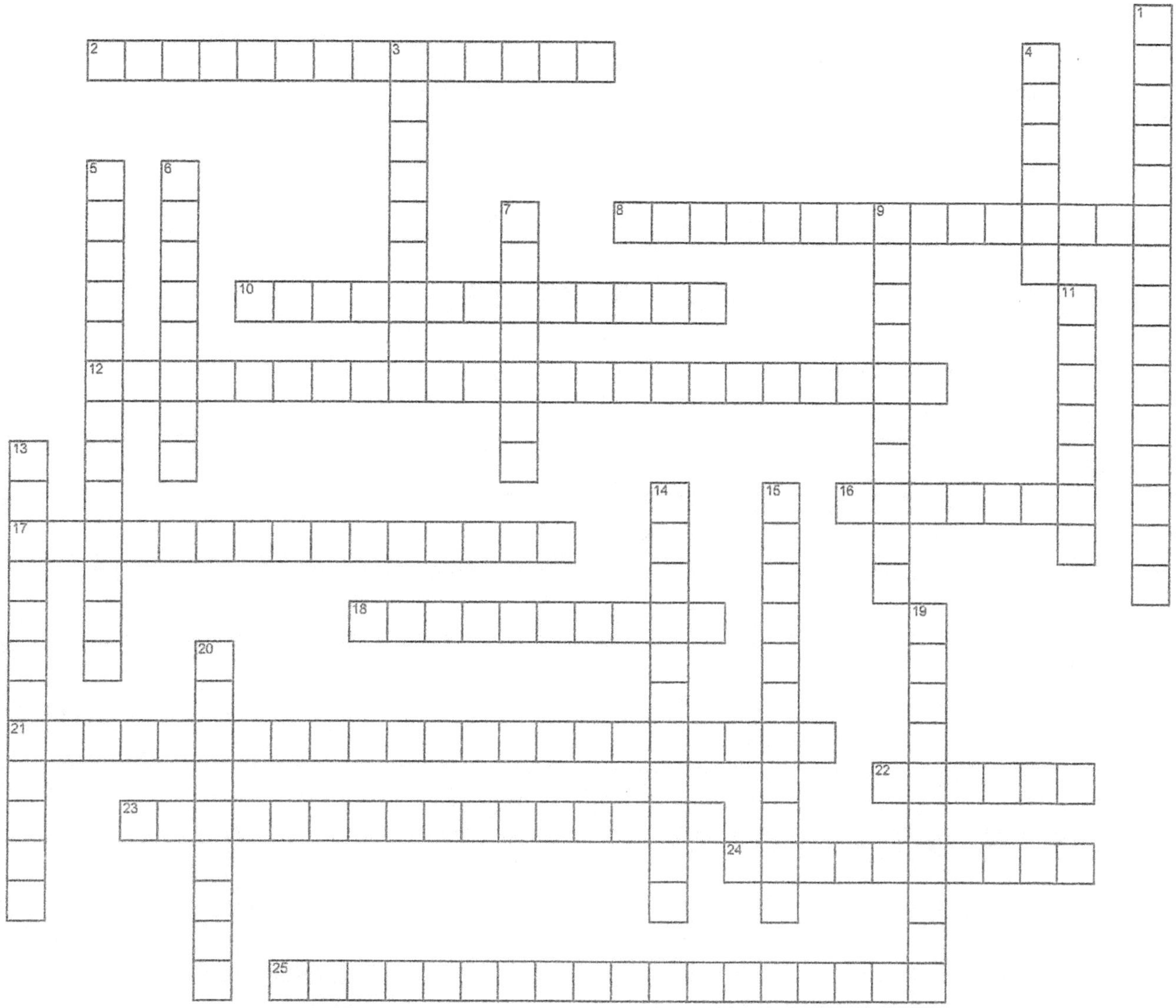

1
2
3
4
5
6
7
8
9
10
11
12
13
14
15
16
17
18
19
20
21
22
23
24
25

ACROSS

2 R.O.A. This ratio divides net income after tax, by the average total assets (3 wds)

8 Another term for the Board of Directors (3 wds)

10 This approach to management includes the input of many managers, and is more often seen in larger facilities

12 An obligation recognized when accumulated benefit obligation of pension plan exceeds the fair market value of plan assets (3)

16 This person gives sworn testimony during a court proceeding

17 An item reported on financial statements that impacts operations of a facility. Large capital expenses are kept off the balance sheet through various classification methods. This is used in order to keep a company's debt-to-equity (D/E) and leverage ratios low. Operating leases are the most common type... (3 wds)

18 Type of survey (also called the federal follow-up survey) done by federal surveyors to verify findings by state surveyors. CMS selects a sampling of state surveys to examine. If federal findings are different than state, federal results prevail.

21 A.Q.L. The actual percentage of goods in a lot of incoming materials that a facility will allow to be defective and still accept the lot (3 wds)

22 Type of communication used by staff to supervisor.

23 Each Medicare patient is eligible for ___ inpatient psyche days. (3 wds)

24 A quality indicator or measure that provides a description of a resident or patient at a given point

25 When the employer is held responsible for the acts of employees within the scope of their employment (2 wds)

DOWN

1 In 1932, this act (also called the Anti-Injunction Act) limited the power of Federal courts to side with management through issuing injunctions (or court decrees) that limited or stopped union efforts to picket, boycott, or strike. Also, yellow dog contracts were banned. (2 wds)

3 Activities which enhance sensory stimuli through music, art, pet therapy, etc

4 Medicare Part B pays ____ percent for medical expenses (physician services, inpatient/ outpatient, labs, therapy, ambulance services, and x-rays), outpatient hospital care, and home health care

5 A restricted fund, which contains a portfolio of marketable securities or other assets donated to an organization, or purchased by donated cash, with the stipulation by the donor that the assets are held permanently for the purpose of producing income to supplement operating revenues. Only the income from these assets may be used. (2 wds)

6 A guarantee concerning goods or services

7 Type of warranty that guarantees a products quality, that is not expressed in a purchase contract. It says that the item sold can perform the function that it is designed for.

9 For each period of illness, a Medicare patient must pay ____ percent of the total expense for his or her hospital stay, during days 61-90. (2 wds)

11 Type of warranty that includes specific promises by the seller

13 P.M. This is the ratio of income to sales. For gross, the formula is gross profit divided by sales. For net, the formula is net income after tax, divided by sales (2 wds)

14 This dilates blood vessels

15 All journals have ____ bookkeeping. (2 wds)

19 Decisions by management on the rate of pay for staff, the amount of discretion supervisors may use in setting salaries the spread between pay rates for long-time and new employees, and the periods between pay raises (2 wds)

20 This test evaluates the strategic impact of an acquisition or business venture on a facility's financial standing (2 wds)

PUZZLE # 22

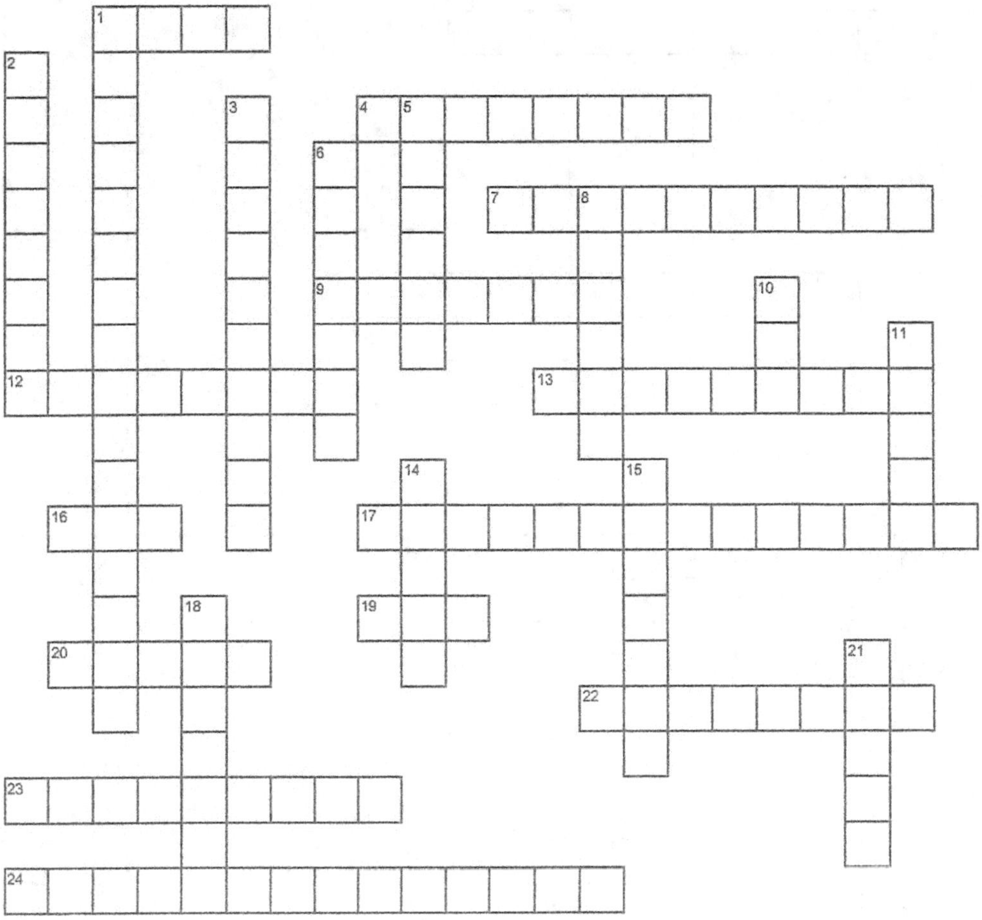

ACROSS

1 This carries blood to the heart
4 "ung"
7 A legal obligation of care, performance or observance to safeguard others rights (3 wds)
9 "cf"
12 Condition when the body cannot metabolize glucose, due to a hormone called insulin.
13 The capacity of an organization to give care
16 Assisted Living Facility (abbreviation)
17 This ratio measures the return the facility earned on funds invested in it. The formula is net income divided by investor's equity (3 wds)
19 Twenty-five percent of the knowledge in healthcare will be obsolete in ___ years
20 This organization provides criminal and civil enforcement tools and funding to fight healthcare fraud. It also mandates a coordinated national healthcare fraud and abuse control program (5 init.)
22 Common stock with a long history of dividend payments and earnings (2 wds)
23 He stated that certain behaviors, such as common courtesy, fall under the category of "a blinding flash of the obvious" (2 wds)
24 This emphasizes the importance of each person being accountable to only one supervisor (3 wds)

DOWN

1 A technique to measure performance through the operating budget. A comparison of actual versus budgeted monetary and volume values at the end of each month (2 wds)
2 Described one who has a physical or mental impairment that limits one or more major life tasks.
3 The amount the resident pays toward nursing facility care (gross income minus allowable deductions) (2 wds)
5 The amount earned from sources other than sales. In a for-profit facility, revenue minus expenses.
6 To test for diabetes, one may measure daily fasting blood sugar levels, or measure the amount of ___ in the urine.
8 The percent of residents who have a condition that is treated as a medical condition that requires special care in rehab is ____
10 Computer-Automated Tomography scan (abbreviation)
11 This goes on the left side of the journal account. A positive amount means an increase in assets and a decrease in liabilities. A negative amount means a decrease in capital and revenue, and an increase in expenses
14 When are locks permitted on resident room doors?
15 ___ tests are conducted on fire alarms, fire doors, smoke detectors, and emergency power generators
18 A legal term for unlawful touching or force without consent. A violation of another's physical integrity
21 For each period of illness, a Medicare patient must pay ___ percent of his or her hospital stay costs during days 91-150

PUZZLE # 23

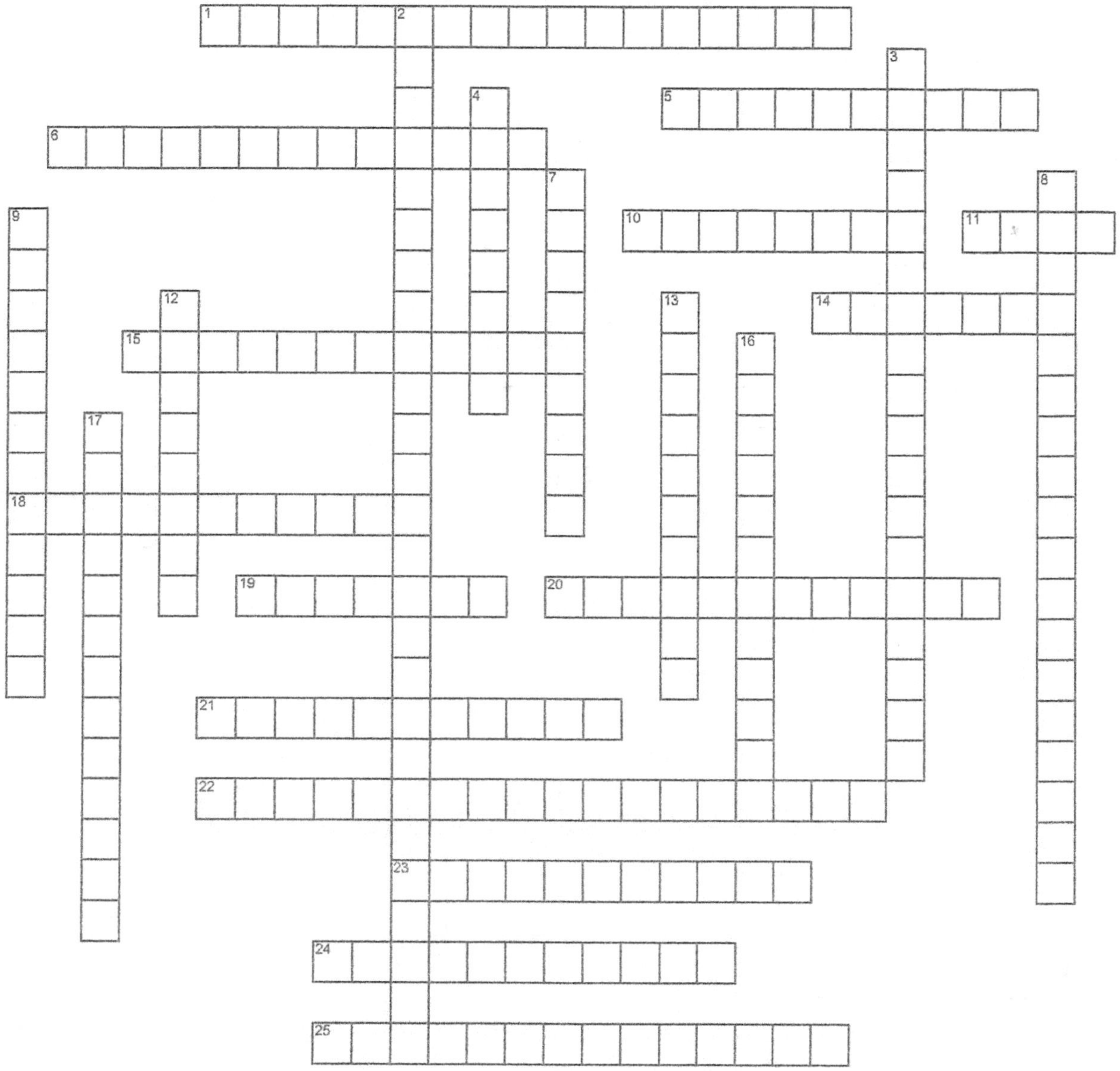

ACROSS

1 The extent that a selection tool measures a trait or behavior perceived as important to a job (2 wds)

5 This deals with material inventories, emphasizing the elimination of all waste, and continual improvement of the production process. (3 wds)

6 The process of giving employees increased roles in the decision-making process in a facility. (2 wds)

10 According to the NFPA, knee clearance under tables, sinks, and work surfaces must be ___ inches

11 True or false: Different employees should complete all of the following tasks: signing checks to pay bills; entering payables into an accounting program; sending out checks to vendors; and reconciling the checking account

14 This person stated "The future will change our plans", regarding the planning process

15 The concept that, whenever in doubt regarding the value of an asset or realization of a gain, an accountant should estimate conservatively, by selecting the accounting procedure which produces the lowest net income (or less favorable financial position)

18 The geographic area from which applicants are to be recruited (2 wds)

19 These remove waste material from the bloodstream, and regulate the amount of body fluids

20 The Medical Director is responsible for the implementation of resident care policies, and the _____ of all medical care.

21 A doctor who specializes in disease and/or injury to bones, muscles, joints and tendons

22 This shows major transactions that occur over the period covered by two balance sheets. It shows how working capital was used during that time. (3 wds)

23 This term, coined by Kriegal, refers to pleasure in the job causing perfection in the work. If employees are happy with their job, it will show in their high quality of work. (3 wds)

24 The importance of an accounting error or omission in financial statements

25 Any asset held as an investment, that can be easily and quickly converted to cash (such as bonds, or easily sold stock) (2 wds)

DOWN

2 R.T.M. (3 wds)

3 If there is a medication error, the first person who should be informed is the ____ (2 wds)

4 This creates job descriptions and specifications (such as skills or qualifications needed to do a job) for all positions within a facility.

7 In 1960, this Act was an amendment to the Social Security Act, to provide medical assistance to the aged (MAA) (2 wds)

8 Also called total quality management, this phrase means that responsibility of quality falls on the employees who deliver the service or product. It can take five to ten years for implementation in a facility. It includes employee empowerment, use of teams, and the use of individual responsibilities for services (4 wds)

9 In 1926, this Act was the first federal legislation sanctioning union organization and the right to bargain collectively with management (2 wds)

12 This establishes the value of a job by comparing it to all the other jobs to be accomplished by an organization (2 wds)

13 Residents should alwasy be within ___ feet of the nearest exit sign (2 wds)

16 The power or legal right to hear and rule on a case

17 The process or assessing and rating all jobs in an organization as a basis for the wage and salary system (2 wds)

PUZZLE # 24

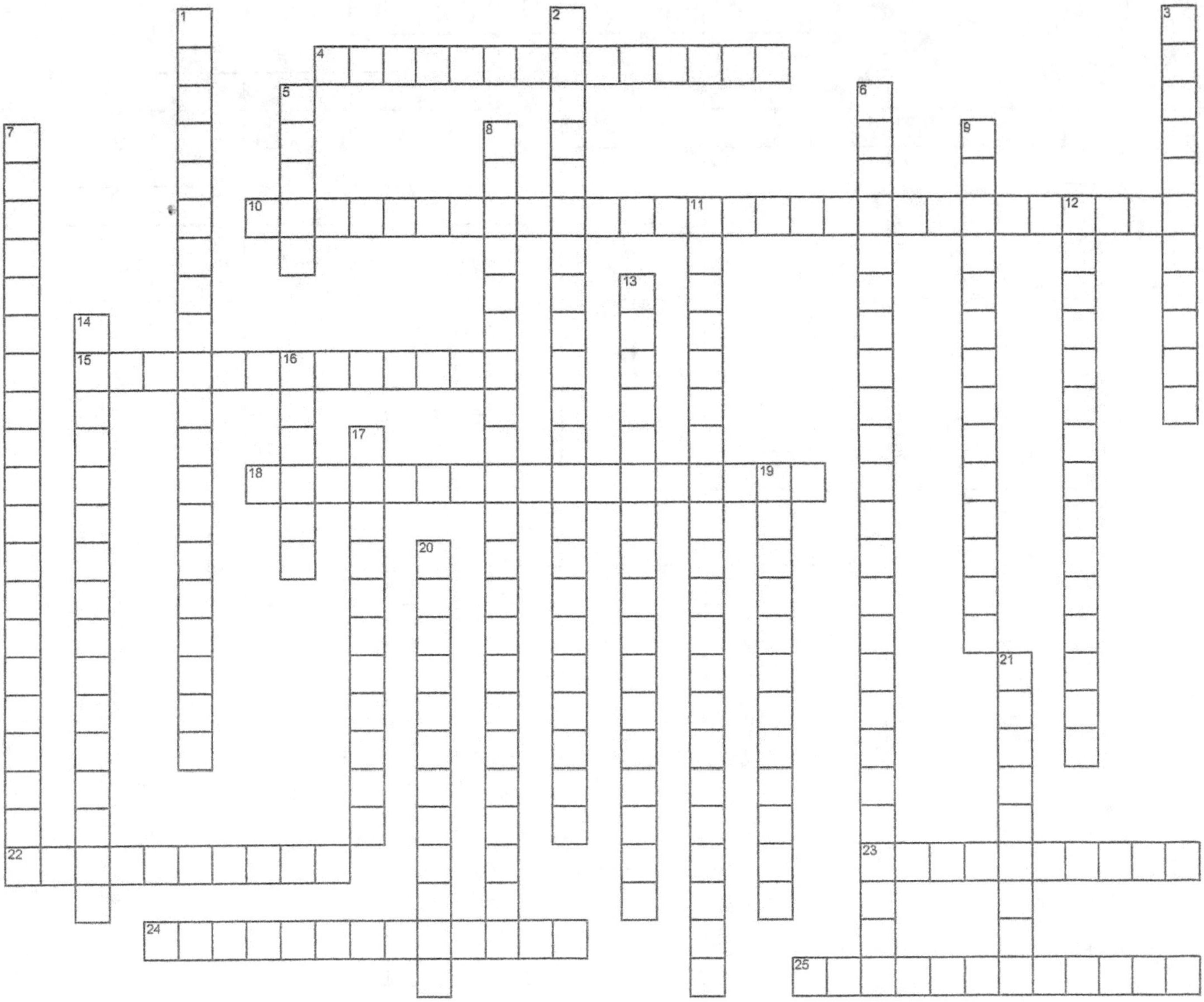

ACROSS

4 A piece of paper that indicates money owed to or by a facility. (example: bank statement)

10 R.A.I. Mandated since 1991 by CMS, this has three parts, including an MDS, CAT's, and a care plan.

15 Part of the operational budget that lists anticipated expenses for the coming year. (2 wds)

18 In 1973, this Act stated that no facility could receive federal funds through acts of discrimination on the basis of physical or mental handicaps. A facility is only allowed to deny an admission if they cannot provide adequate services (2 wds)

22 A dentist who extracts teeth

23 A "good" or "easy" death. A non-accidental termination of life.

24 Someone with this disease will produce little or no urine (3 wds)

25 Also called the Statement of Financial Condition/ Position. This financial document provides a measure of net worth, and shows what a company owns and owes. It is a "snapshot" of fiscal health at any one specific time. (2 wds)

DOWN

1 F.I. Private healthcare insurers that serve as federal government agents in the administration of the Medicare program, including the payment of claims. They do reimbursement reviews and medical coverage reviews. (2 wds)

2 When blood is backed up in the circulatory system, which causes fluids to leak from the bloodstream. (3 wds)

3 This induces coughing and secretions

5 "t.i.d." means ___ times a day

6 O.I.G. They can impose monetary penalties, and exclude providers that violate the False Claims Act from participating in Medicare, etc. They investigate violations of the Anti-Kickback Statute. Their concerns are reducing fraud and abuse in federal healthcare programs. (4 wds)

7 Principle that states if inclusion or omission of disclosure would influence the decision of a reasonable person, it should be disclosed (2 wds)

8 When blood pressure decreases upon standing (2 wds)

9 A federal survey, within fourteen days of a standard survey, regarding substandard care issues (2 wds)

11 A written summary of non-compliance with regulations found during a survey or complaint investigation (3 wds)

12 This person serves as the liason with local health officials (2 wds)

13 Type of journal that records payments made for services and supplies used for resident care, and all other operations of a facility (2 wds)

14 Establishing wage rates for jobs, by comparing all jobs in the organization to a touchstone job in the facility (3 wds)

16 Type of power where employees and residents agree that the Administrator is skilled and knowledgeable.

17 A doctor who specializes in x-rays, MRI's and CAT scans.

19 This established fundamental United States law.

20 Theory that employees seek an exchange where their wages and benefits are equal to their work effort (especially when compared to co-workers) (2 wds)

21 The pay variation permitted within a class or grade of jobs (2 wds)

PUZZLE # 25

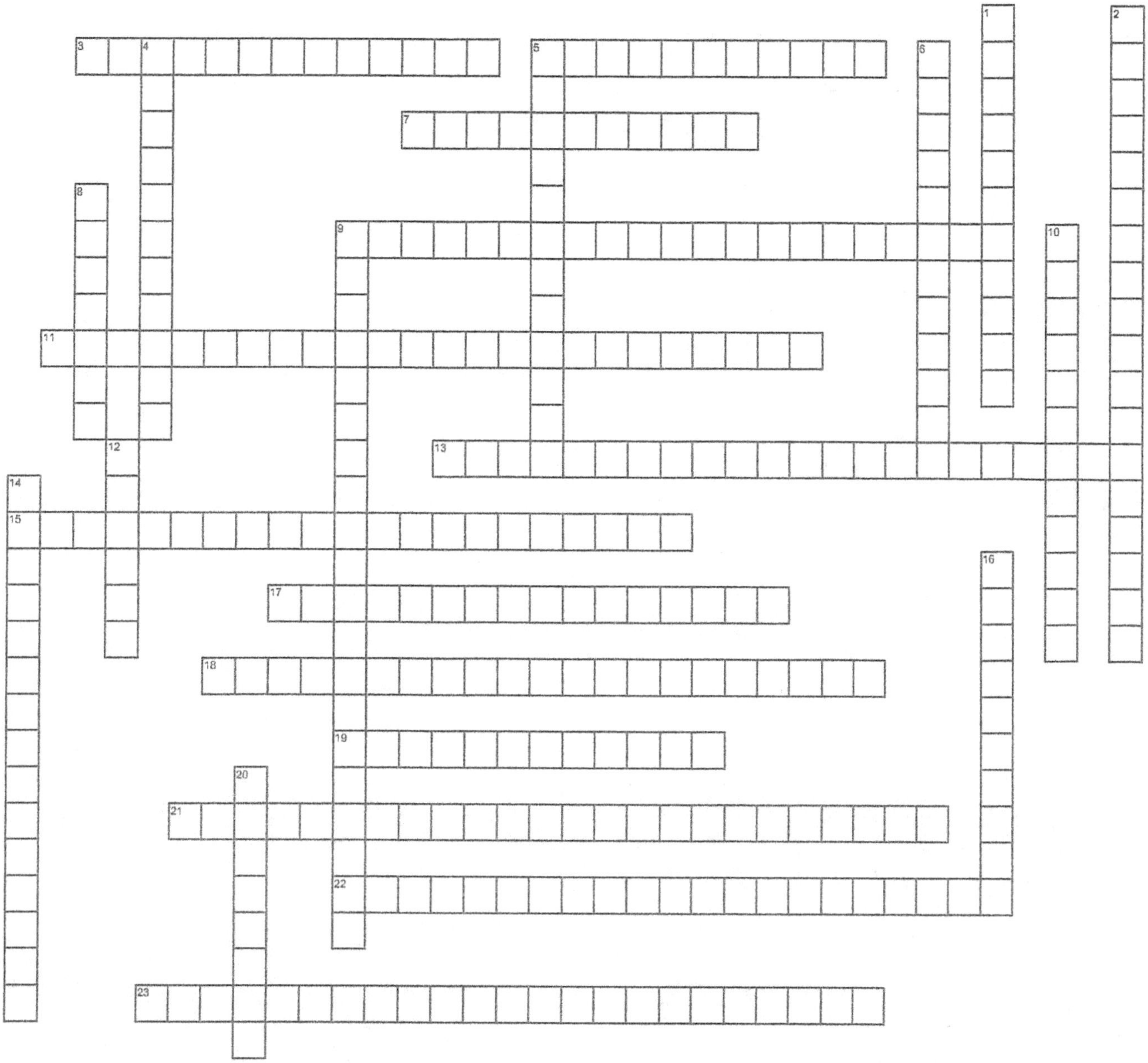

ACROSS

3 When employees and/or other private people sue a facility on behalf of the government, for fraud committed against the government. (They may receive 10-25% of the recovery in successful suits) (3 wds)

5 Those who are systematic, thorough, and are known to ask detailed questions are said to be _____ (2 wds)

7 When a defendant is formally charged with an offense.

9 Adaptations which allow a resident to stand independently, transfer alone, and participate in activities (2 wds)

11 I.P.M. A program of Serv Safe that outlines procedures for controlling access of pests in a facility (3 wds)

13 In 1914, an Act that established the FTC, and gave the FTC responsibility for promoting free and fair competition in interstate commerce in the interest of the public through: the prevention of price fixing agreements, boycotts, combinations in restraints of trade, unfair acts of competition, and unfair or deceptive acts and practices (3 wds)

15 Blood (2 wds)

17 The diffusion of authority, responsibility and decision-making power through different levels of a company

18 The overall style or atmosphere of a facility. It dictates how people relate to each other. (2 wds)

19 Those who are intuitive, quick, and use a simple approach to decision-making are said to be ____. (2 wds)

21 The most accurate way to count supplies used, and those remaining (3 wds)

22 To combat home care fraud, the DHHS (Department of Health and Human Services) enforced this initiative, targeted at home health agencies, nursing facilities and durable equipment suppliers (3 wds)

23 The study and diagnosis of what is perceived to be a problem that is adversely affecting a nursing facility (2 wds)

DOWN

1 These items contact, but do not penetrate skin (example: blood pressure cuff)

2 In 1938, an Act that was amended many times, but whose focuses were minimum wage, overtime, child labor and equal rights for hourly employees. Also stated that overtime could be calculated two weeks at a time. (3 wds)

4 Managing for quality includes quality planning, quality control and quality ____.

5 Type of leadership that permits subordinates to make decisions and function within limits defined by managers. (2 wds)

6 A counter demand by a defendant against the plaintiff (which is independent of the original claim) (2 wds)

8 Type of contract that is established when a need arises, and then terminated after the need has been met. (2 wds)

9 Offering one service for all markets (2 wds)

10 These items touch mucous membranes (examples: razor, thermometer)

12 A right granted in exchange for an agreed upon sum to buy or sell property.

14 This includes all planned revenues by source, and all anticipated expenses by "natural classification", such as salaries and wages, supplies, utilities, taxes, interest and depreciation (2 wds)

16 OMN. NOC. (2 wds)

20 These items enter sterile tissue or the vascular system, or through that which blood flows (examples: needles, catheters)

PUZZLE # 26

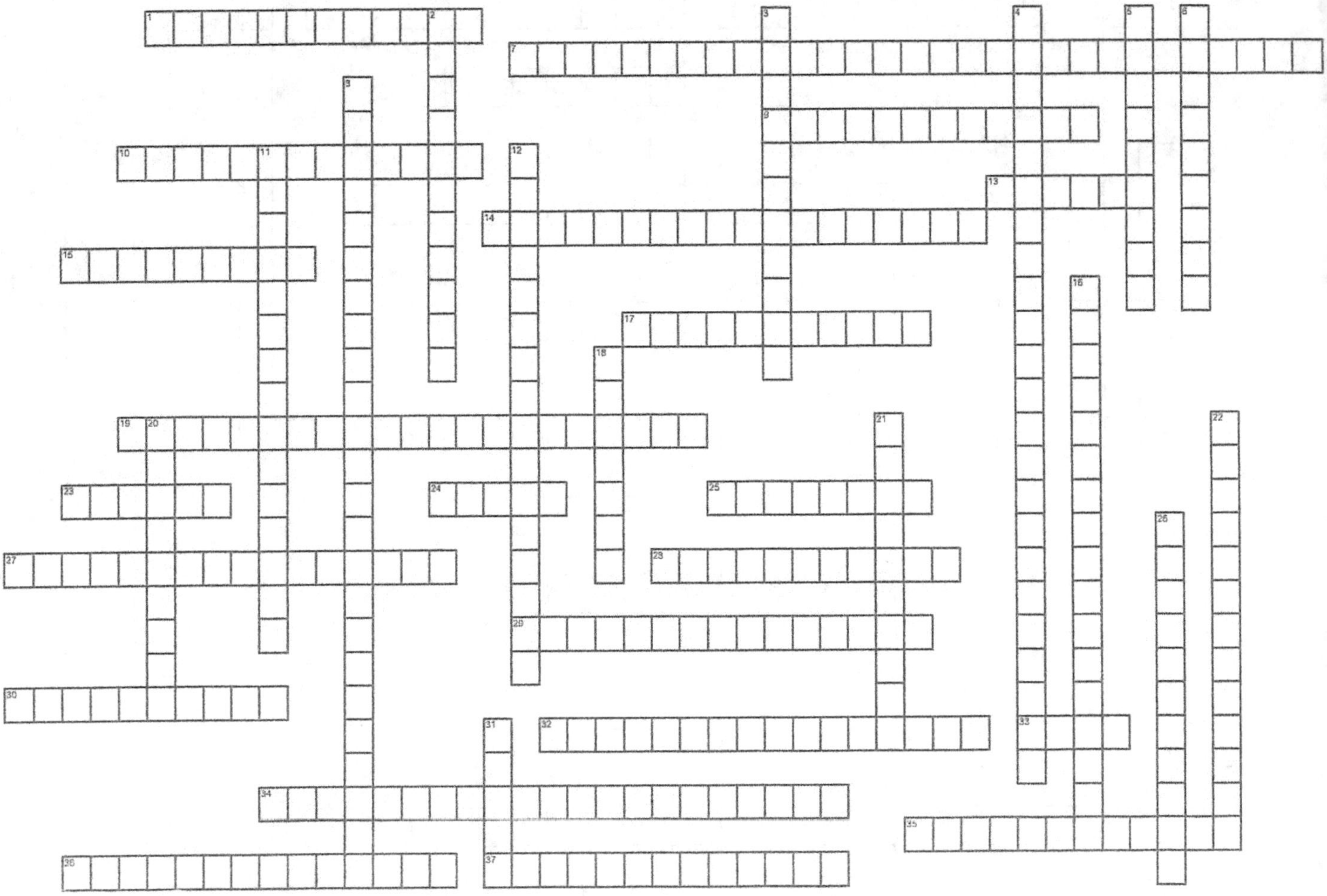

ACROSS

1 Type of leadership that permits subordinates to make decisions and function within limits defined by managers. (2 wds)
7 The sale of receivables as a means of short-term financing. (The seller transfers receivables and the risk of default) (4 wds)
9 A counter demand by a defendant against the plaintiff (which is independent of the original claim) (2 wds)
10 A written order to arrest someone (written by a judge in that jurisdiction) (2 wds)
13 Kriegal stated that 100% effort required when short-staffed leads to job dissatisfaction. It is better to aim for a passionate ___ %.
14 In 1938, an Act that was amended many times, but whose focuses were minimum wage, overtime, child labor and equal rights for hourly employees. Also stated that overtime could be calculated two weeks at a time. (3 wds)
15 An unsecured bond
17 Symptoms include painful urination and blood in the urine
19 To combat home care fraud, the DHHS (Department of Health and Human Services) enforced this initiative, targeted at home health agencies, nursing facilities and durable equipment suppliers (3 wds)
23 This type of power has to do with inducing or persuading employees or residents. If an Administrator is unable to induce or persuade, then certain approvals may be withheld
24 Level of management where a licensed person is responsible for formulating and enforcing policies for the entire facility. Also equivalent to "origination"
25 As a managerial behavior, deciding what needs to be done, setting short and long term objectives, and figuring out how to achieve them. (also known as "forethought).
27 A statement of skills, education and experience required for a job. (2 wds)
28 Managing for quality includes quality planning, quality control and quality ____.
29 This includes all planned revenues by source, and all anticipated expenses by "natural classification", such as salaries and wages, supplies, utilities, taxes, interest and depreciation (2 wds)
30 Type of business transaction at market-established prices, between two unrelated parties (2 wds)
32 This describes the role, and code of conduct for nurses (3 wds)
33 In general, all organizations seek to ___
34 Blood (2 wds)
35 Those who are intuitive, quick, and use a simple approach to decision-making are said to be ____. (2 wds)
36 An original record containing details to substantiate a transaction entered into an accounting system (examples: purchase order, receipt, invoice) (2 wds)
37 This helps identify trends in many measures of financial performance by comparing the same ratio over several periods. (To be most useful, ratios should be compared with industry averages over a period of time) (2 wds)

DOWN

2 This is used to evaluate the extent of which an employee meets a trait or requirement for a job (2 wds)
3 These items contact, but do not penetrate skin (example: blood pressure cuff)
4 The study and diagnosis of what is perceived to be a problem that is adversely affecting a nursing facility (2 wds)
5 What percent of facilities have a resident council? (2 wds)
6 This staff member is federally required to be full time, and is responsible for maintaining all medical records (2 wds)
8 The most accurate way to count supplies used, and those remaining (3 wds)
11 Another term for "Medical Nutritional Therapy" (2 wds)
12 This states how a deficiency during a state survey will be corrected, what actions the facility will take to prevent reoccurrence, and the time frame for corrections (3 wds)
16 A registered nurse who meets additional state requirements (2 wds)
18 This ratio measures a company's ability to meet short-term debt obligations. As a rule, a ratio greater than 1.5 indicates that a company has a good short-term financial strength.
20 This model of care is a patient-centered, holistic approach, that promotes mental, emotional, spiritual, social and physical healing
21 A legal term describing where a case is taken, if the defendant pleads not guilty to a felony or misdemeanor. Here is where plea bargaining begins, in order to reach an agreed upon disposition. If no disposition is reached, the case is adjourned, motions are made, and more bargaining ensues.
22 A company whose ownership shares are not publicly traded (2 wds)
26 When a defendant is formally charged with an offense.
31 The CMS database that lists facility information and survey results. (Online Survey/ Certification and Reporting) (5 initials)

PUZZLE # 27

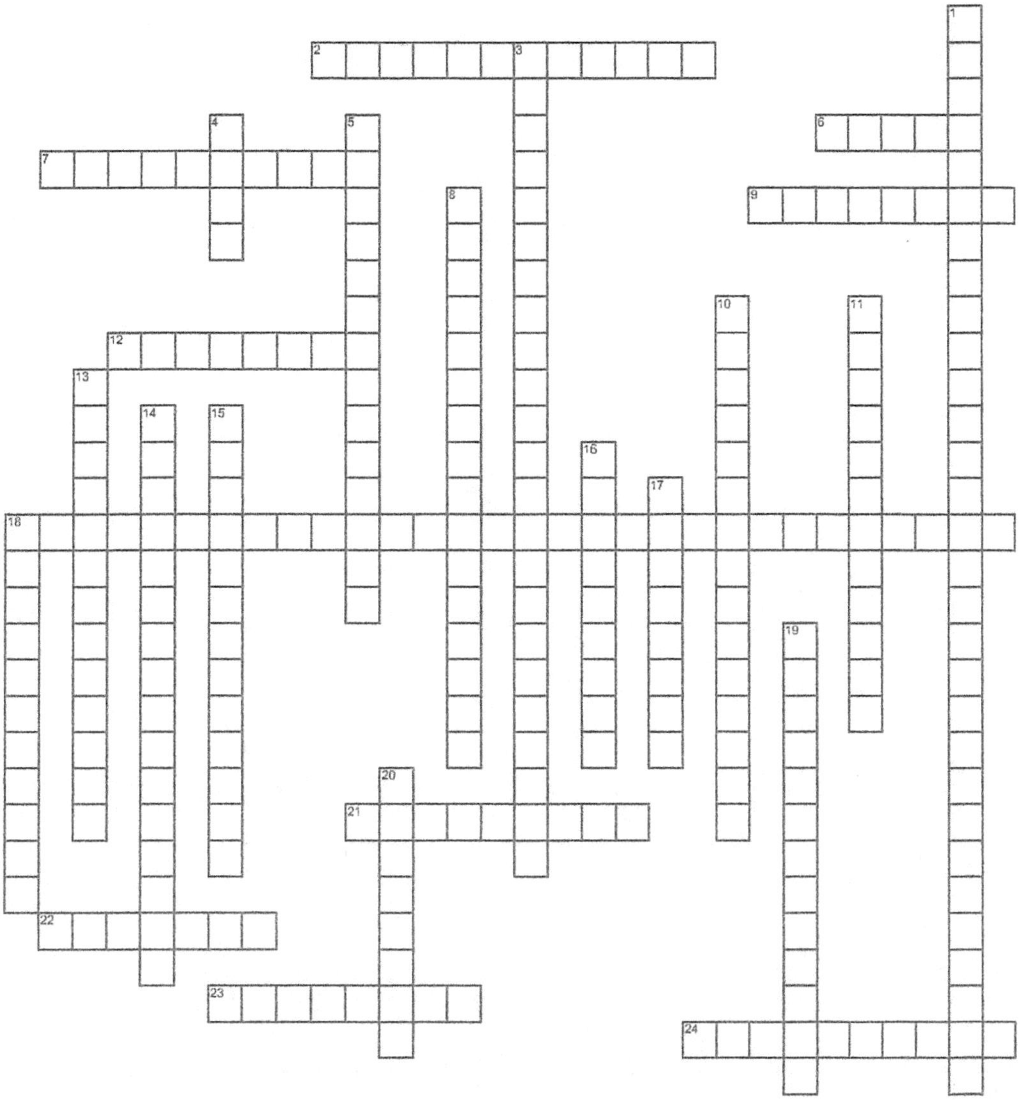

1
2
3
4
5
6
7
8
9
10
11
12
13
14
15
16
17
18
19
20
21
22
23
24

ACROSS

2 Also called general fund; also called operating fund. Type of fund for assets which may be used at the discretion of the governing board, to carry out the purposes for which the organization was founded
6 When a patient is given a chemical restraint, he or she must be monitored hourly for the first ___ hours
7 Type of audit that determines if a facility is meeting specific rules and regulations
9 Enforced by the EEOC in 1963, this Act states that an employer must pay the same wage to a male or female worker in the same job. Pay must equal skill, effort, and responsibility. (2 wds)
12 Type of audit where a financial representative studies the financial records of a facility to ensure that it meets facility policies
18 This states that history is made or measurably influenced by people who become leaders (5 wds)
21 Regarding Medicaid, the percent of money spent on institutionalized care over the past two decades has slightly _____
22 When a patient is given a chemical restraint, he or she must be monitored continuously for the first ___ minutes (30 minutes for nonparenteral)
23 This requires the forecasting of economic, social and political environments anticipated for an organization, and the resources that will be available
24 Type of audit that examines the efficiency of administration

DOWN

1 In 1974, this Act required firms with more than ten thousand dollars in federal contracts to have affirmative action programs for the employment and advancement of Vietnam Vets. (4 wds)
3 R.O.I.C. This shows how well a facility used its funds over a long period of time. The formula is net income divided by (non-current liabilities plus owners equity) (4 wds)
4 Number of years most states require that medical records are maintained
5 The Standards for Privacy of Individually Identifiable Health Information includes guidelines issued by the Department of Health and Human Services to protect the rights of patients by keeping their ______ private (2 wds)
8 A revision to an organization's capital structure. It may involve the exchange of debt obligations for equity interests, or exchange of one type of debt for another
10 System which is comprised of bones, muscle, cartilage, tendons, and joints (things used to move)
11 Inputs, processor, outputs and control (2 wds)
13 This report is done monthly, by the bookkeeper, and it calculates the total routine charge for each resident or service recipient (2 wds)
14 Translating goals into clear policies, identifying appropriate measures, stating limits to deviation, getting information to staff members, stating policies of action to be taken, taking corrective action, renewing quality measures, finding control measures that are functional and valued by the staff, and knowing limitations and/or capabilities of the system, are all steps of ____ (3 wds)
15 They adapt written by-laws that describe an organization's structure, and establish authority and responsibility. (2 wds)
16 "Q.H." (2 wds)
17 G.P. The formula is pay rate multiplied by regular hours, plus overtime rate multiplied by overtime hours (2 wds)
18 Setting objectives to be achieved by an employee before the next performance appraisal (2 wds)
19 Type of leadership where the leader dictates policies and procedures, decides goals, and directs/ controls all activities, with very little participation from subordinates
20 This is a government health insurance program that is state-run

PUZZLE # 28

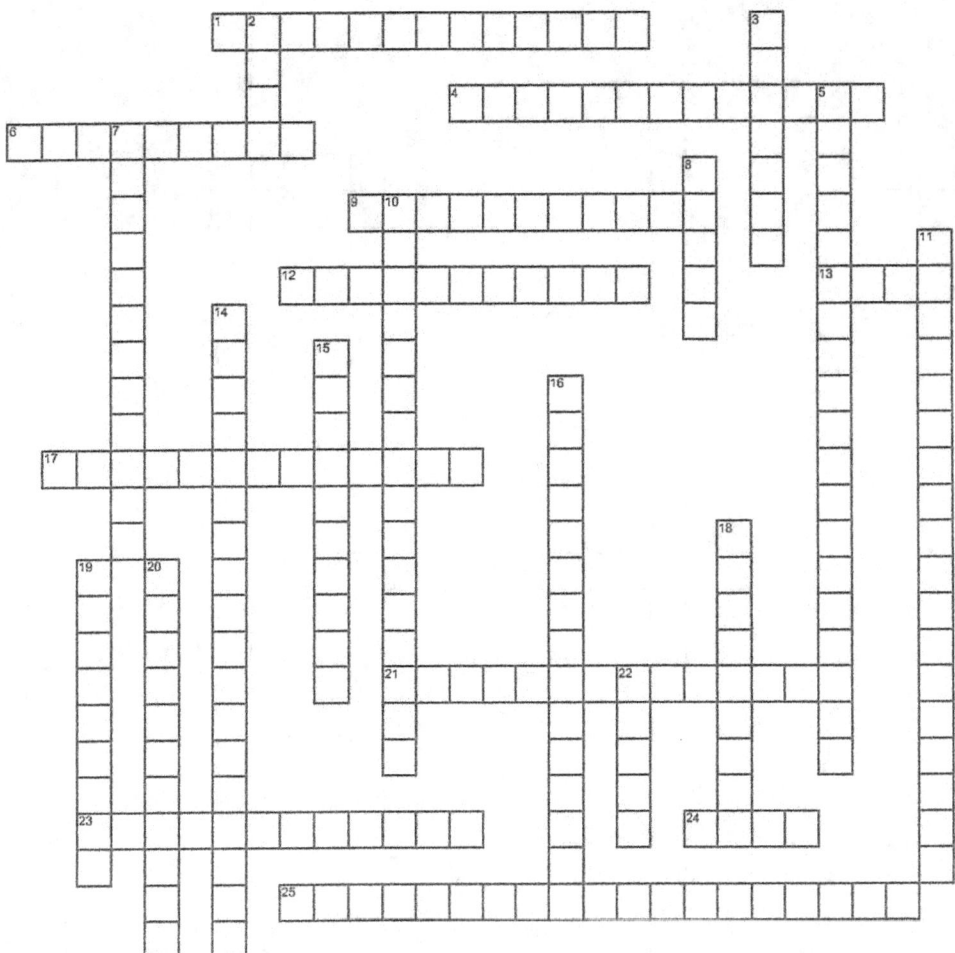

1
2
3
4
5
6
7
8
9
10
11
12
13
14
15
16
17
18
19
20
21
22
23
24
25

ACROSS

1 Type of assessment completed within 14 days of admission. Uses RAI's (Resident Assessment Instruments). Each team member must sign, and certify its accuracy. Done at least every 12 months
4 The coordinator of the infection prevention and control program is called the infection ____.
6 Chemical restraints must be ordered by a ____ in writing, including the dose, frequency and duration of the medication
9 A form of negligence, where an unlawful or improper act is performed
12 This type of inventory includes identifying competition for personnel, estimates in-migration/ out-migration of workers and looks at wage scales in the area. (2 wds)
13 True or false: Personal fraud on a comprehensive assessment can be charged with up to $1000.00 fine. Making another employee commit fraud can result in up to $5000.00 fine
17 Borrowing funds through interest-bearing instruments (2 wds)
21 The four categories for violations under OSHA are: small (no fine), non-serious (where there is a direct correlation between the condition and health), serious (a major fine may be charged) and _____ (this can close a facility) (2 wds)
23 The annual percent of income earned on an investment (3 wds)
24 On an MDS, quality indicators are listed in what color?
25 Total patient days in a year, divided by the number of admissions in a year is the formula for ____. (4 wds)

DOWN

2 Omnibus Budget Reconciliation Act (also called the Nursing Home Reform Act) This Act made changes to the Social Security Act, including reforms to Medicare and Medicaid (4 initials)
3 For Medicaid patients, patient care costs are billed _____, with one composite bill for all Medicaid residents
5 A publication from 1987 by four federal agencies, setting standards by which federal agencies determine the acceptability of validation procedures used for written tests and other selection devices. It is called the uniform guidelines on employee ______(2 wds)
7 Costs which vary disproportionately with volume
8 Number of years that Virginia requires medical records to be maintained
10 Term referring to how a person may not recover from an injury that they receive when they voluntarily expose themselves to a known danger (3 wds)
11 Used to improve the evaluation of training efforts, these are also called behavioral objectives (2 wds)
14 Copying errors in cell divisions make cells that are unrecognizable to the body, which triggers the immune system to attack. This is called the ___ theory of aging. (2 wds)
15 Emergency orders for chemical restraints are good for ____ hours (2 wds)
16 The person who signs and certified the completion of a comprehensive assessment (2 wds)
18 Type of audit where an independent CPA examines financial records and gives an opinion
19 Source of law that emanates from federal and state legislatures
20 This type of principle calls for deferring recognition of revenue until that revenue is earned (2 wds)
22 OSHA citations are issued at the end of an inspection, or by mail. Citations must be posted for ___ days, or the duration of violation, whichever is longer

PUZZLE # 29

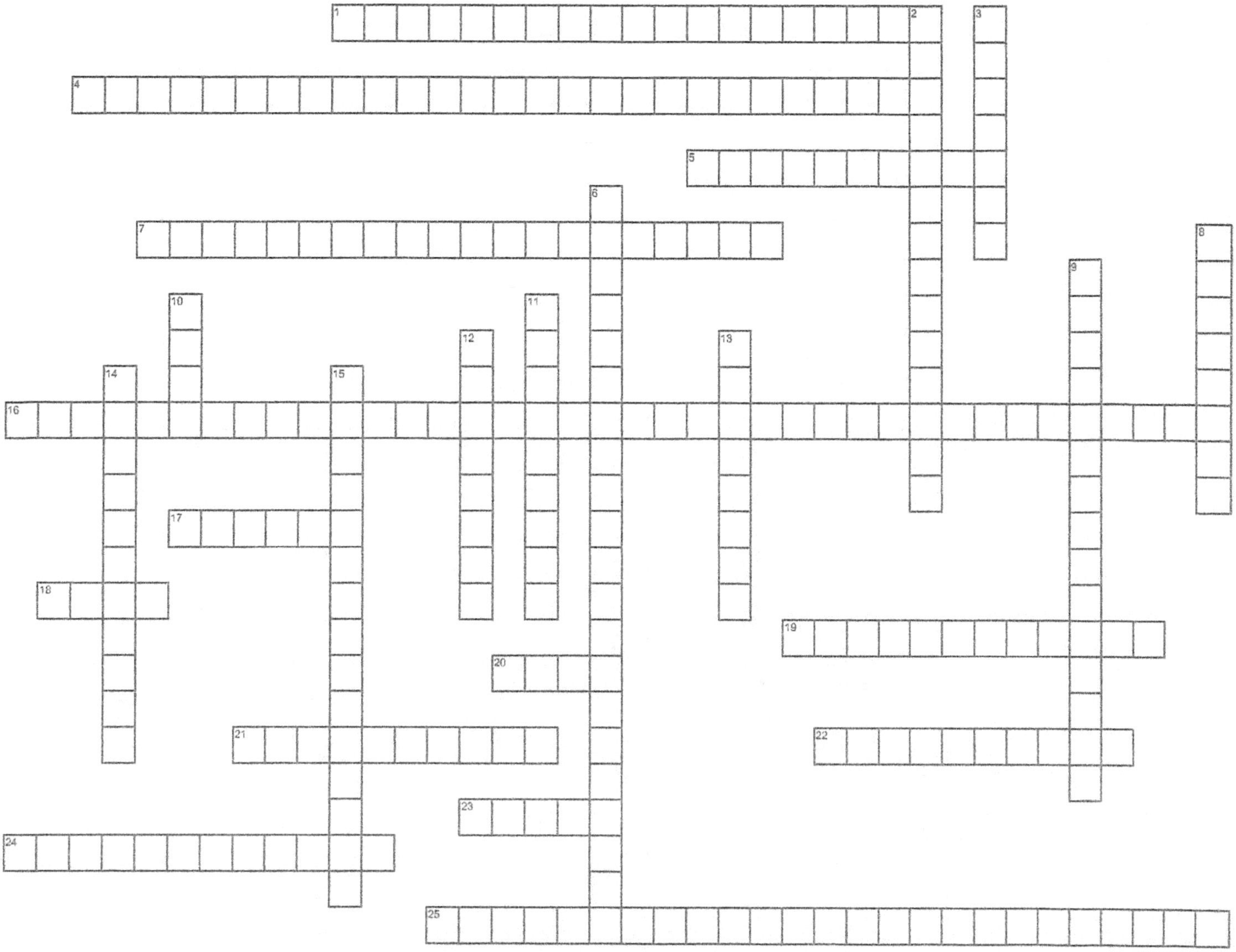

ACROSS

1 Symptoms of this condition include itchy, dry skin, mental confusion, weakness, muscle cramps, nausea, and diarrhea (3 wds)
4 P.P.E. (3 wds)
5 Type of power given to a particular person; associated with a persons position in an organization
7 This phrase refers to those with needed skills being able to negotiate higher wages (2 wds)
16 P.A.S.R.R. (also P.A.S.A.R.R.) (Used for residents with mental illness or mental retardation) (5 wds)
17 The most recent full (or quarterly) assessment when quality measure scores are calculated
18 Type of life insurance that has no cash value, and no dividends. Costs less than other types of life insurance.
19 Doctor who diagnoses and treats heart diseases
20 How one will move from point A to point B, in order to put one's strategy to action
21 Patients are considered "skilled" care if they are assigned to one of the ____ of 53 highest RUG groups in the initial MDS assessment (2 wds)
22 A flexible line of progression through which an employee moves during their employment with an organization. Also called a career ladder. (2 wds)
23 A federally required screening on all nursing home residents, prior to admission, to determine if a resident has M.I. or M.R. (5 initials)
24 Every page of a medical record which is faxed must be marked _____
25 In the 1960's, CMS developed these health and safety standards. (3 wds)

DOWN

2 Symptoms of movement disorders, antipsychotics or metabolic disease. (examples: tremors, rigid movements, tics, blinking, pacing)
3 A defined way to do a task. Strict parameters on how a strategy is performed
6 Term for the digestive system (2 wds)
8 Regarding substandard care, four elements are required for a civil suit. They are _____, breach or violation of contract, damage or injury, and causation (2 wds)
9 The degree that a test, interview procedure, or other selection tool measures the skills, knowledge or performance requirements of a job (2 wds)
10 A small number of people committed to a common purpose, with a set of performance goals which they are mutually accountable for
11 Any medical record being faxed must include a ____ (2 wds)
12 A solution to move from where one is, to where one wants to be
13 The principle that money is the basic measuring unit for financial reporting
14 In 1947, an Act that placed limits on unions (amended in 1974 to include Nursing Facilities and hospitals). It restored the rights of managers to express their views regarding unions and unionizing efforts. Managers were then free to express opinions about their employee's voting for a union in the workplace. (2 wds)
15 In 1973, an Act that required federal government contractors to mount affirmative action programs for the handicapped. (2 wds)

PUZZLE # 30

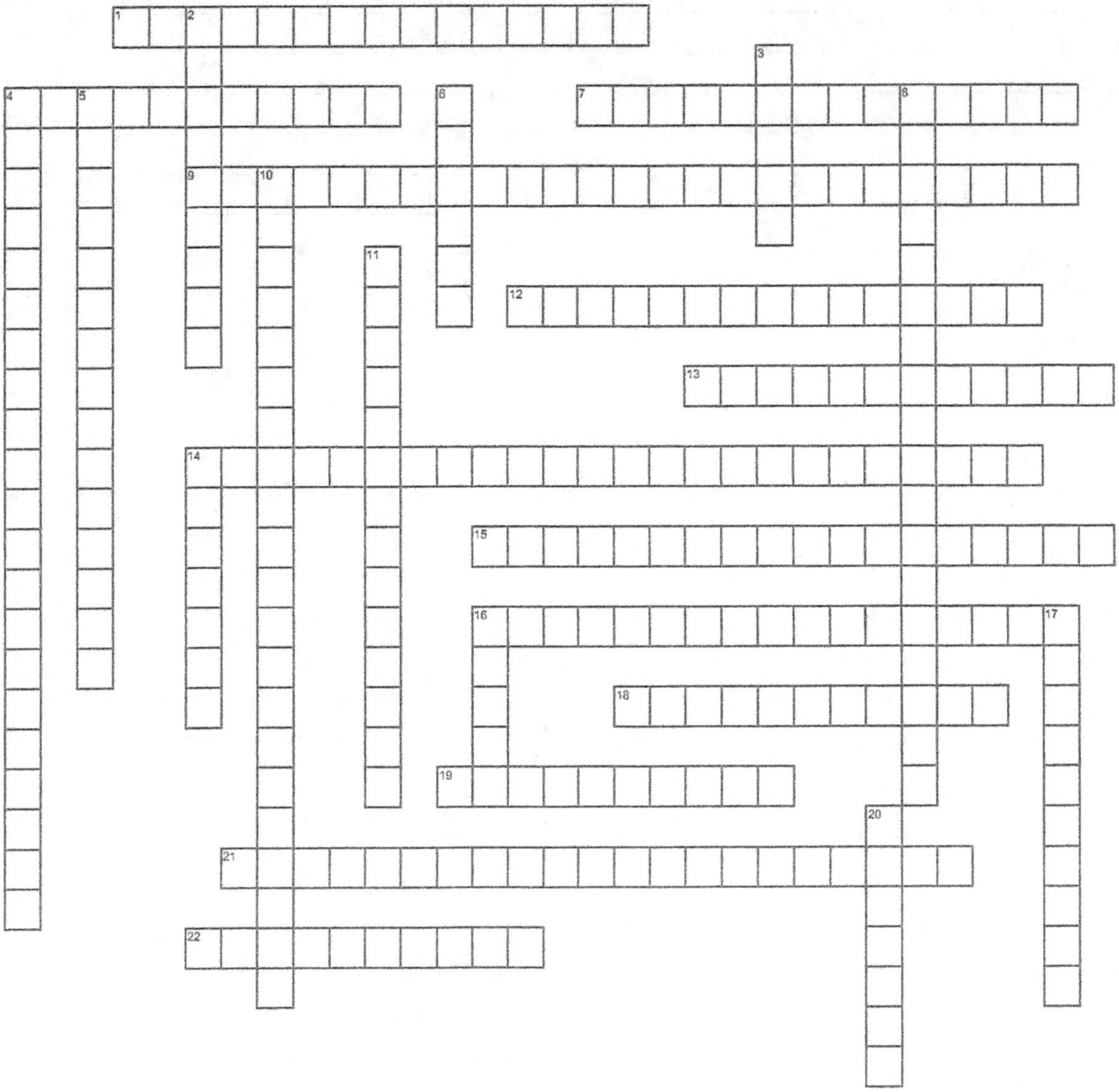

ACROSS

1 A published register that lists the requirements for long-term care facilities (regulations for Medicare and Medicaid) (2 wds)

4 Type of test that evaluates strategic impact of acquisition or start-up of a new business venture. (The cost of entering must not exceed future projects) (3 wds)

7 Also called the circulatory system. Powered by the heart, this system circulates blood. When cell health deteriorates, it is usually due to a decreased effectiveness of this system, which interferes with the supply of nutrients to the cells.

9 I.D.R. Regarding a state survey, regulations allow for an I.D.R. and appeals process. (3 wds)

12 F.I.F.O. For inventory costing... In case of deflation, older and less expensive supplies are used first. Higher-priced goods remain in inventory longer (4 wds)

13 An inpatient program for a resident who has had an acute event, has a determined course of treatment, and does not require extensive procedures (2 wds)

14 In 1968, an Act that limits the amount of an employee's earnings that may be garnished, and protects employees from being discharged for any one indebtness (3 wds)

15 The maximum loan amount based on a percentage of the borrowing facility's appraised value (4 wds)

16 Symptoms from anti-psychotics, including head jerking, mouth movements, and tongue thrusting disorders. (2 wds)

18 Awareness activities which build self-esteem. (examples: delivering mail, folding laundry, resident council)

19 S.W.O.T. includes strengths, ____, opportunities and threats.

21 R.T. (2 wds)

22 Medicare allows ____ hours for an examination of a resident after admission (2 wds)

DOWN

2 Defining the terms "leading" and "deciding" are often quite ____

3 Level of management that a charge nurse is a member of

4 The ability to issue orders to subordinates in an organization. (3 wds)

5 When one is subject to liability without fault. It is applied when the activity is so dangerous to others that public policy demands absolute responsibility on the part of the wrongdoer (2 wds)

6 A serious crime, punishable by imprisonment in a state or federal penitentiary for more than one year

8 Intentional neglect, causing pain or suffering to an infirm, aged person (4 wds)

10 F.M.L.A. In 1993, this Act stated that companies with fifty or more employees must allow up to twelve weeks of unpaid leave-of-absence to employees who have spent twelve or more months on the job. (reasons for leave-of-absence may be pregnancy, childbirth, adoption, serious illness, etc). Those twelve months on the job do not have to be consecutive. Employee must give a thirty-day notice before LOA. (4 wds)

11 The process of studying a procedure or business in order to identify its goals and purposes and create systems and procedures that will achieve them in an efficient way. Equally useful to the Administrator, Director of Nursing, and Housekeeping Manager. (2 wds)

14 An organization that pays Medicare claims submitted by doctors and other medical suppliers. Deals with claims from doctors who are covered under Medicare Part B.

16 The care of a subacute resident costs ___ times that of a typical patient

17 An impartial person chosen by both parties of an argument to decide the issue

20 A state survey must be conducted nine- ___ months from the previous survey

PUZZLE # 31

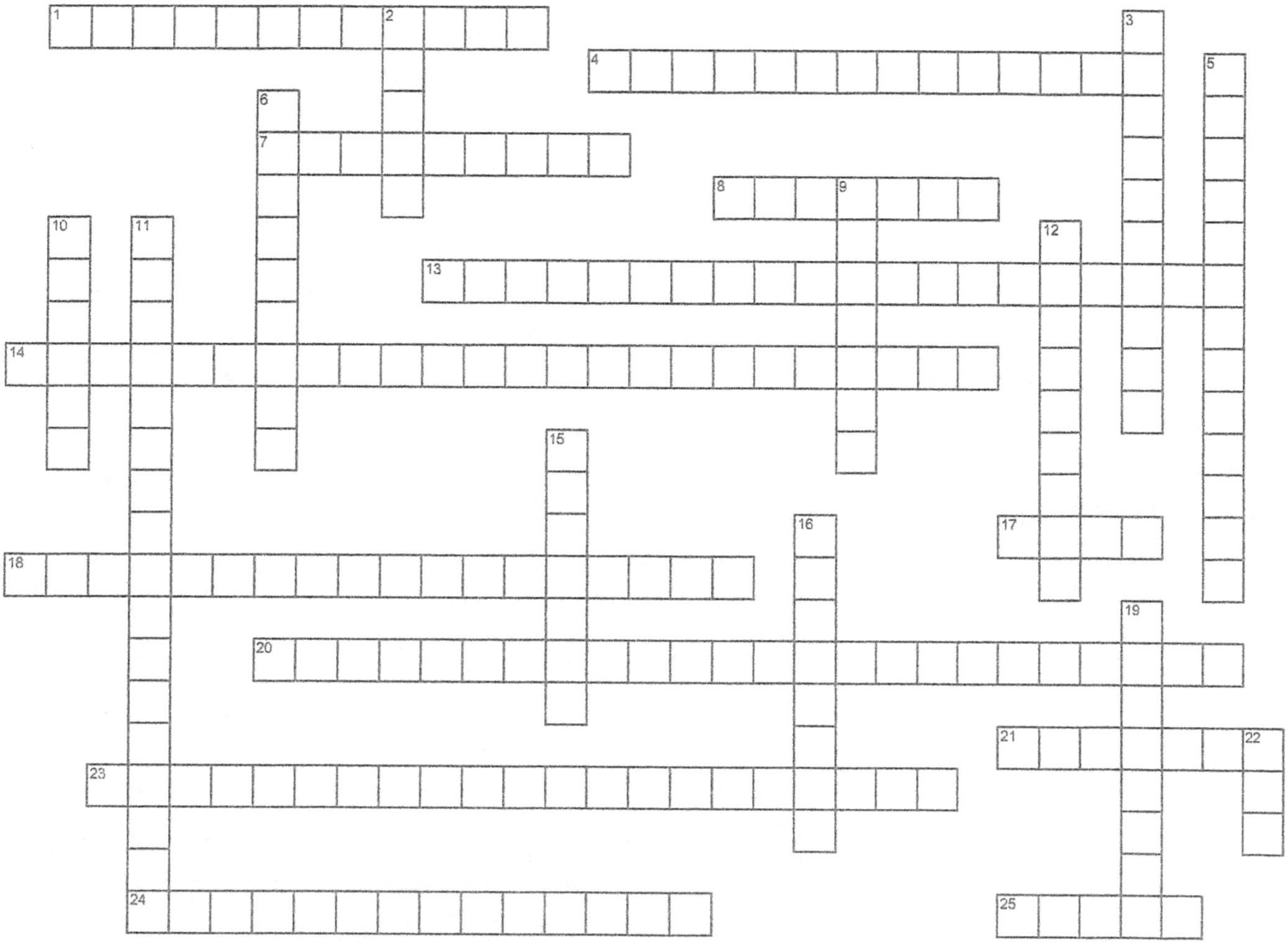

ACROSS

1 The beginning inventory, plus purchases made minus the amount used equals _____ (2 wds)

4 The duty to have and use ones degree of knowledge and skill usually possessed by able, similar healthcare providers in similar events (3 wds)

7 A doctor who specializes in the prodecures and treatments of nonsurgical cases

8 The primary structural component of the human body is _____.

13 Elements that give a facility an edge (2 wds)

14 Those who are interested, and have the necessary funds, access and quality (in other words, those who meet the requirements for 24-hour nursing care in a nursing facility) (3 wds)

17 True or false: A 401k (also known as an employee retirement plan, or a salary-reduction plan) is not taxed.

18 The main area of concern in dietary, from 1993-2006 was _____ (2 wds)

20 C.F.R. Federal requirements and guidelines for surveyors (4 wds)

21 Inventory balances are recorded ___ on the balance sheet

23 The federal government has identified ____ diseases reimbursable to hospitals for Medicare patients (4 wds)

24 Five responsibilities in this department are planning, organizing, staffing, directing/ leading, and controlling (2 wds)

25 End inventory represents an ___ in an organization

DOWN

2 Extinguisher used to treat trash, wood, paper, or plastic fires (2 wds)

3 Type of leadership where members of a group participate in the decision-making process. Usually very effective, with high productivity and better morale. Also called participative leadership

5 This ratio measures a company's investment potential, or how much a share is worth per dollar of earnings. The formula is market price per common share divided by primary earnings per common share (2 wds)

6 Who is responsible for initial and annual dietary assessments?

9 When an employee dislikes work, prefers extensive direction, does not want responsibility, and has little ambition. Type of administration, based on the belief that managers should use fear and/or punishment to motivate employees, who must be closely watched. (by Douglas McGregor, a management theorist) (2 wds)

10 Term meaning "by law" (2 wds)

11 This results in better care for residents (2 wds)

12 A company's merchandise intended for sale in the normal course of business

15 How many hours are permitted between dinner and breakfast, if a night time snack is provided?

16 How many hours are permitted between dinner and breakfast, if no night time snack is provided?

19 What temperature (in degrees, Fahrenheit) must cold food be kept at, or below? (2 wds)

22 Was there relative stability in healthcare during the 1970's and 1980's?

PUZZLE # 32

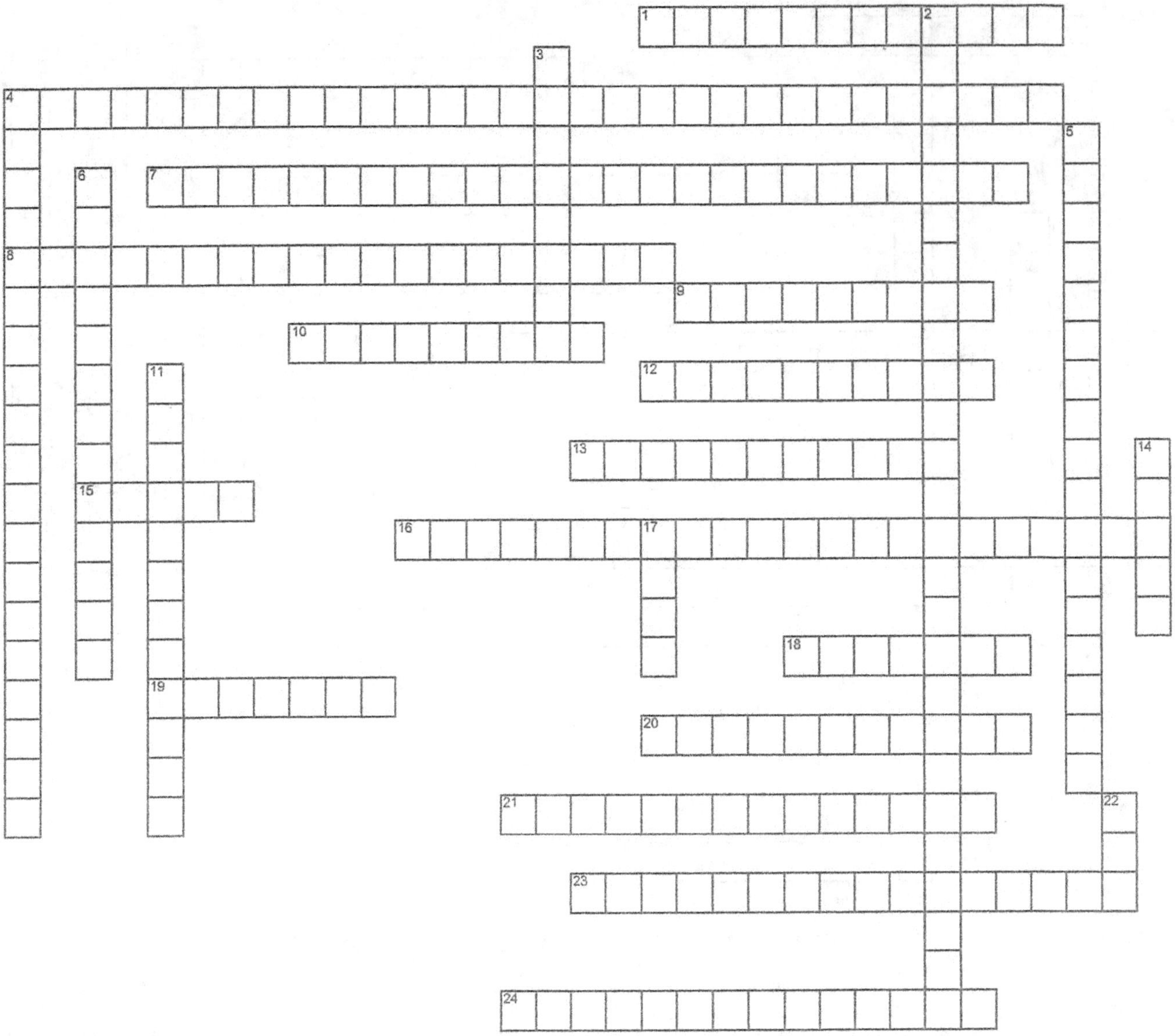

1
2
3
4
5
6
7
8
9
10
11
12
13
14
15
16
17
18
19
20
21
22
23
24

ACROSS

1 There are ____ disease codes in the International Classification of Diseases (2 wds)

4 This designates the annual dollar amount an employer contributes to a pension plan. THe employer makes no guarantee of future benefits beyond the value of the money set aside in the pension fund each year. (4 wds)

7 Pension benefits that an employee receives when he retires (based on years of service and compensation level); specific benefits promised. (4 wds)

8 Rules issued by the Department of Labor, which outline requirements of healthcare facilities in preventing the spread of infections. (Must be used when providing care to all residents) (2 wds)

9 Since 2013, all facilities must have a _____ system installed.

10 Buying a stock, currency or commodity in one market, and selling it in another market at the same time. Taking advantage of price differences between two markets. (buy low, sell high)

12 A promissory note with no set maturity date. Holder can require payment at any time. (2 wds)

13 Type of leadership referring to when decisions must be made quickly, and there is no time to solicit input from others

15 Extinguisher used to treat liquid fires (from cooking oil, gas, kerosene, or paint) (2 wds)

16 D.R.G.

18 This type of administration states that managers must come up with new strategies to keep employees motivated. It states the importance of a satisfactory quality of life, and includes that which is covered by theory Y. (by Douglas McGregor, a management theorist) (2 wds)

19 The opposite of theory X. This type of administration states that employees are self-motivated and have great self control. (by Douglas McGregor, a management theorist) (2 wds)

20 This induces perspiration

21 In 1959, this Act protected the interests of an individual union member against possible union abuses. Also called the Labor-Management Reporting and Disclosure Act (2 wds)

23 An often misunderstood process used by managers to make decisions. Imprecise process. (2 wds)

24 Who is responsible for quarterly dietary assessments? (2 wds)

DOWN

2 S.S.I. Ensures minimal monthly income to needy, and is administered by the local Social Security office (3 wds)

3 Finding the right person for each well-defined job. This is a management function, not a broad personnel search

4 This ratio is used by leaders to judge the credit=worthiness of an entity. The formula is projected annual cash flow divided by the required annual debt payments (3 wds)

5 A.A.A. They assist elderly, by bringing their homes to minimum standards and providing added security to reduce break-ins (4 wds)

6 A facility culture where staff consult with residents, and show empathy in making decisions. Residents accommodate staff most of the time, but have some choice regarding routines and/or options. (2 wds)

11 Restores the injured party's financial situation to match the party's financial state before suffering harm. These are damages recovered for actual injury or economic loss. Punitive damages are not included.

14 Extinguisher used to treat electrical fires (2 wds)

17 An electric current to stimulate nerves for therapeutic purposes (for example, pain relief). The process involves connecting electrodes to the skin. (Transcutaneous electrical nerve stimulation) (4 initials)

22 Emergency power can have no more than a ___ second delay

PUZZLE # 33

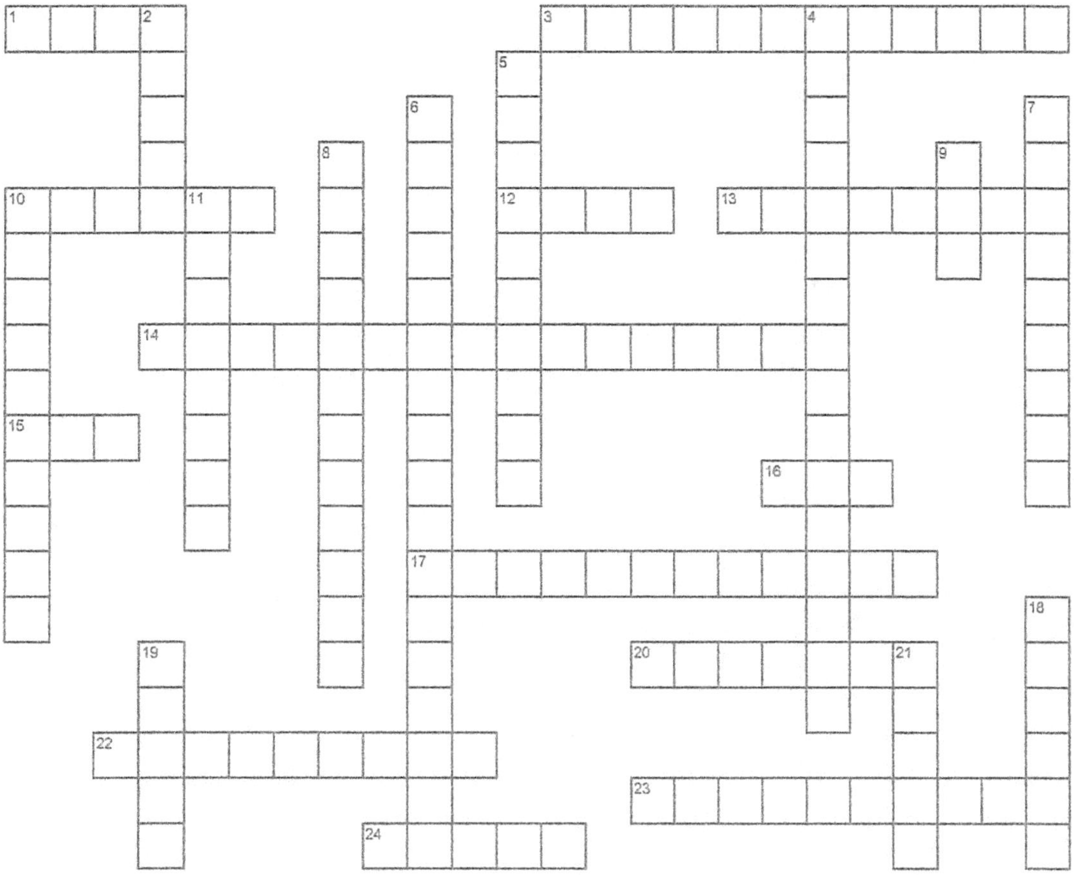

ACROSS

1 This tax is withheld from wages, and helps fund Social Security retirement and Medicare programs. It is matched by the employer. (Quarterly, the employer must file Form 941)
3 A summary score based on the components of an employee performance appraisal (2 wds)
10 A term that means "daily"
12 When one is forced to have sexual intercourse, without consent
13 Removing an uncollectable account from account receivables. (As a result, bad debt expense goes up, and account receivables goes down) (2 wds)
14 OBRA promotes quality of life and ____ care (2 wds)
15 On an MDS, reimbursement level determination items are recorded in what color of ink?
16 This means "as necessary" or "when needed" (3 initials)
17 A system of interactions among the three available inputs: people, materials, and money
20 Money that is rewarded by the court or jury to the person wronged
22 A number of people report to one supervisor, who then have face-to-face interaction, and who have a bit of interdependence in carrying out tasks to achieve organizational goals (2 wds)
23 Letting decisions be made at the lowest possible level.
24 A facility has ____ days from an assessment to encode data and transmit that data to the State.

DOWN

2 An examination of compliance with accounting standards and policies
4 Shareholder's equity consists of invested money and _______ (which are previous profits minus dividends to owners) (2 wds)
5 The person who observes medication passes, and records and reports drug error rates is the consulting ___.
6 This regulates the process for addressing violations of criminal law (such as arrest, arraignment, conference and trial) (2 wds)
7 Approval for building a new facility is sometimes _____ to obtain from government agencies (due in part to zoning and building codes)
8 When probate court appoints a substitute decision-maker for an incompetent patient.
9 A collection of tasks assigned to an employee
10 Type of harassment: A demand for sexual favors, and the adverse employment decision that results from the rejection of those demands (3 wds)
11 An infection associated with institutionalization, which can reoccur.
18 The environment of a facility remains ___ control
19 Type of life insurance that builds cash value (which means it can be converted to cash), and normally pays interest (dividends). Often more costly than other types of life insurance.
21 What level of government determines the policies and requirements for Medicaid?

PUZZLE # 34

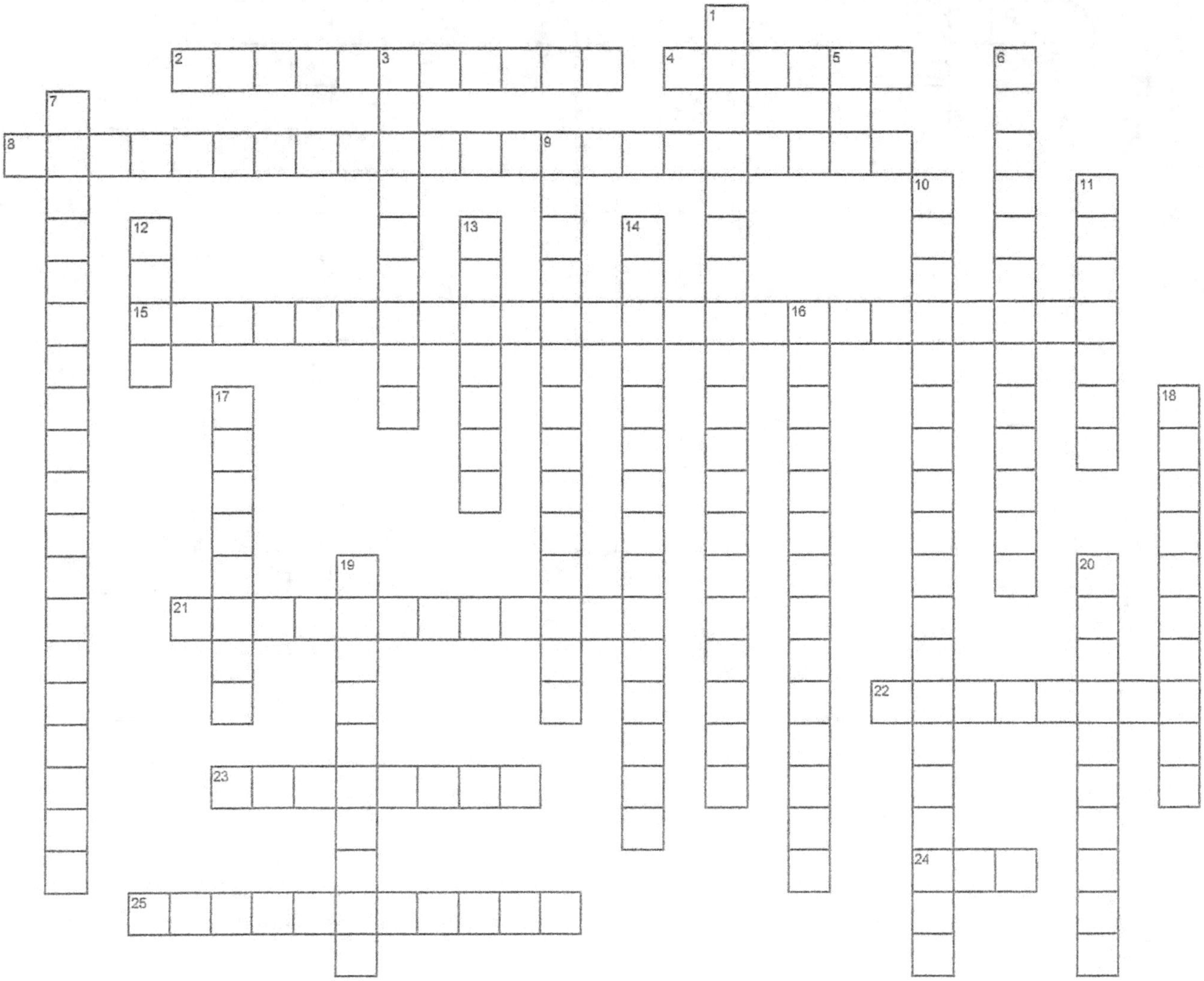

ACROSS

2 The three primary sources of malpractice are failure to obtain effective consent before intervening in the life of a resident, breach or violation of a contract or promise, and _____ care

4 Resident weight loss should not exceed 7.5% in a ___ day period.

8 M.T.M. Measures individual motions (micro-motions) such as reaching, grabbing, and position. (3 wds)

15 M.R.I.

21 Phrase which means "buyer beware". (2 wds)

22 When a facility is cheap, meaning that they are not providing high quality services

23 Resident height should be recorded ____.

24 The National Association of Long-Term Care Administrator Boards. A non-profit agency, comprised of state boards/ agencies who license NF administrators. They provide examinations, publications, and research. (3 initials)

25 If a change in level is between 1/4" and 1/2", it is considered a ______. (2 wds)

DOWN

1 In 2006, an Act that allows payment to relatives to give care to family members, regardless of a patient's age. (3 wds)

3 An advanced directive option must be given to each resident at time of ____

5 Resident weight loss should not exceed ___ percent in 180 days

6 This consists of stock rather than cash, paid to shareholders (2 wds)

7 C.O.W. Nursing homes must enroll in the Clinical Laboratory Improvement Act program by obtaining a _____. The facility pays a certification fee every two years, and follows manufacturers instructions. (3 wds)

9 End of period entries (finance). These entries are recorded to complete the bookkeeping cycle. They record certain expenses to the period (depreciation) and update revenue income, expenses, and losses. (2 wds)

10 Summaries of a nursing facility's financial well-being within a time period (2 wds)

11 Second step in the budgeting process (determining objectives to follow)

12 If there is a change in level over 1/2", it is considered a ____

13 Who certifies that a care plan is complete?

14 Fractions that use the numbers on a financial statement (2 wds)

16 Each fire alarm system must be _______ supervised

17 Rehabilitation = (type of payment, typically)

18 A resident's _____ is considered one of the most reliable indicators of nutritional status in long-term care (2 wds)

19 Fourth step in the budgeting process (estimates cash inflows and outflows for twelve months. Also used to defer non-urgent expenses to a month with high cash inflow) (2 wds)

20 Two methods to allocate indirect costs are step-down and ____.

PUZZLE # 35

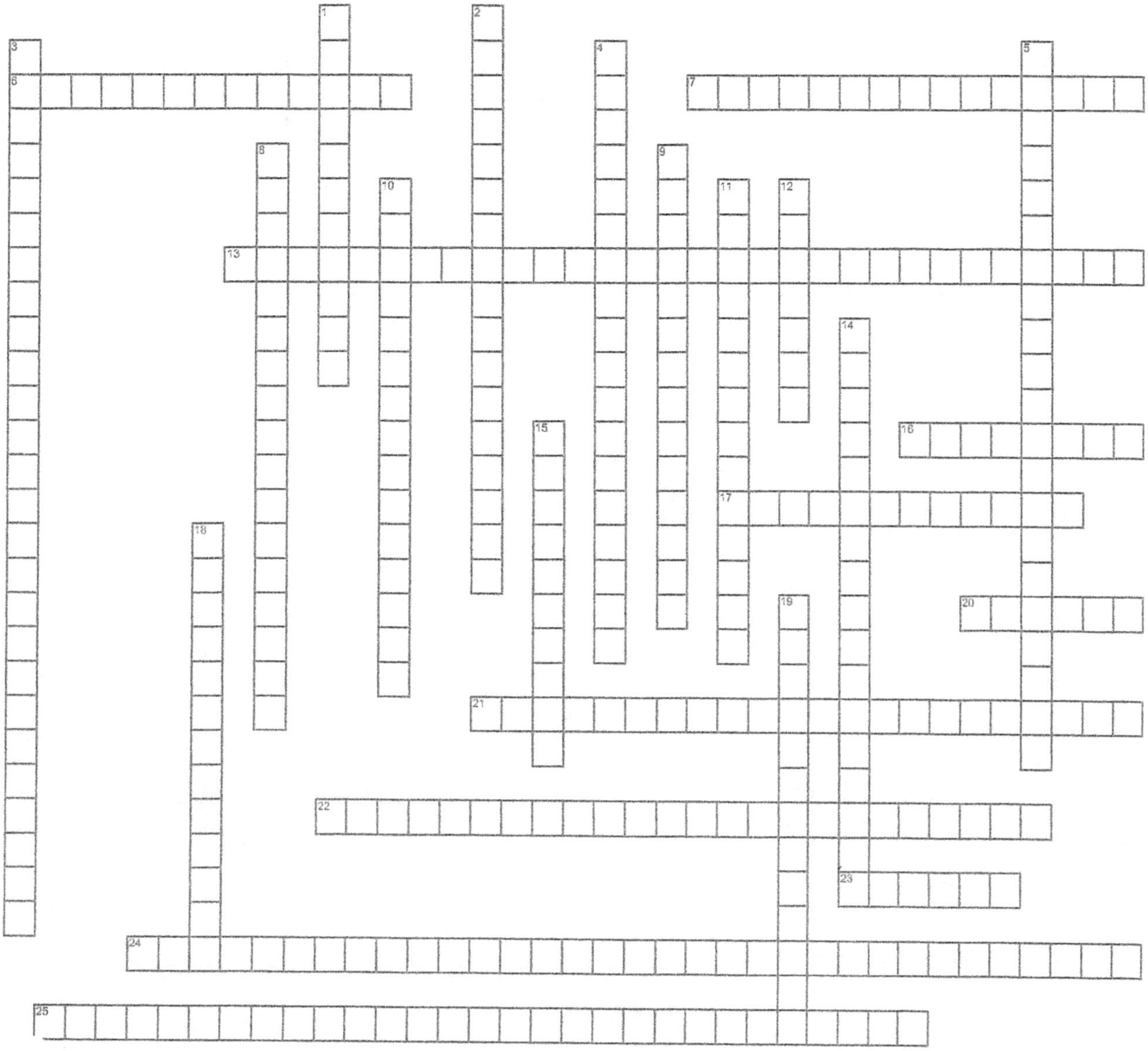

ACROSS

6 AB Costing. Type of costing method that assigns costs to specific areas of the facility (also known as departmental area costing) (2 wds)

7 Care plans include the attending physician but not the ________. (2 wds)

13 In 2001, this Act required employers to choose more safe needle devices, involve employees in identifying and choosing those devices, and maintain a log of injuries related to contaminated sharps. Used to eliminate/ minimize employee exposure (4 wds)

16 Each facility must have a _______ operated fire alarm system

17 On financial reports, must be paid within one year (2 wds)

20 According to the ACA (Affordable Care Act), effective 2015, one is considered full-time if he or she works ___ or more hours per week.

21 S.O.M. The current set of requirements and guidelines given to surveyors (3 wds)

22 A ratio that shows how long it takes for a facility to collect revenue from residents. (4 wds)

23 Handrails must extend ____ inches beyond a ramp or stair, and must be parallel to the ground

24 NFPA. A private, non-profit organization, with more than 150 committees. Not a government agency, no federal requirements. (4 wds)

25 C.L.I.A. Act that established quality standards for all lab testing to ensure accuracy, reliability, and timeliness of patient test results, regardless of where the test is done. (3 wds)

DOWN

1 Assigning all costs (direct or indirect) to cost centers. This yields a picture of the expense of providing each service. This information is used to decide if a service should be continued or discontinued. Only after this is done, can an accurate job of rate setting be completed. (2 wds)

2 The principle that assumes a company will continue to operate in the future (which is important when comparing the value of a running business to one being liquidated). This justifies recording obligations as if they will be paid, and transactions at acquisition cost, rather than at current market value. In other words, preparing financial statements on the assumption that the facility will remain open long enough to carry out and fulfill commitments (2 wds)

3 N.P.I. HIPAA mandated. To improve efficiency and effectiveness of electronic health records and electronic medical records, providers are issued this.(3 wds)

4 In England, a minimum annual income was guaranteed to all. (2 wds)

5 A.D.L. Eating, bathing, dressing, toileting and transferring. These are measured in section G of the MDS. (4 wds)

8 A concept that requires accounting records be prepared with documentable records kept by the facility (such as receipts, bank statements, bills and invoices) (2 wds)

9 Developed by the National Fire Protection Association, this lists fire safety standards (3 wds)

10 Third step in the budgeting process (includes expense budget and revenue budget. Measures performance by variance analysis) (2 wds)

11 This measures the number of days of cash operating expenses a company could cover with its unrestricted cash, cash equivalents and marketable securities on hand. The formula is cash divided by (operating expenses divided by days in a period) (4 wds)

12 Resident weight should be recorded ____.

14 First step in the budgeting process (internal, external) (2 wds)

15 Long-term care= (type of payment, typically) (2 wds)

18 Fifth and final step in the budgeting process (2 wds)

19 Another term for resident-centered care (2 wds)

PUZZLE # 36

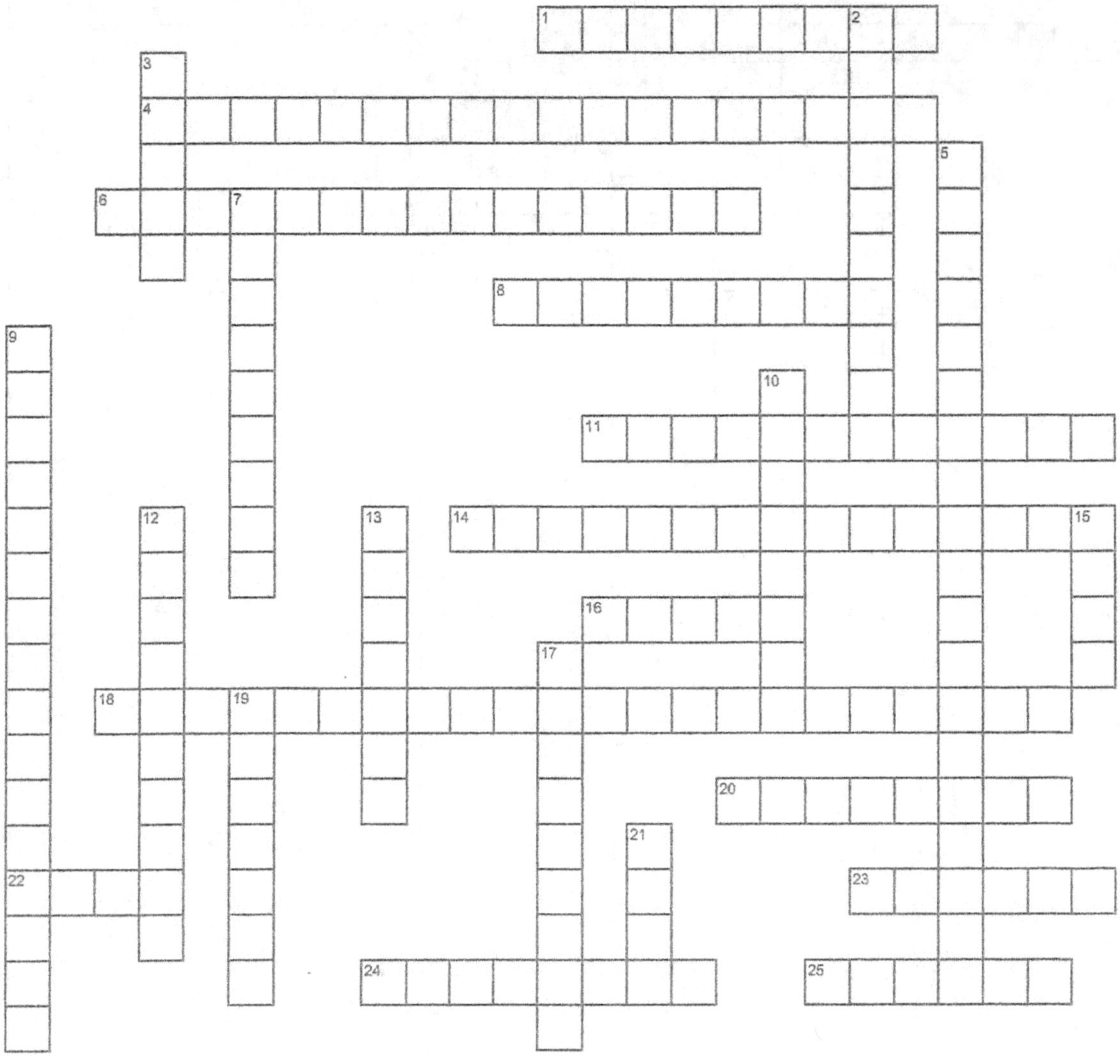

ACROSS

1 Medicaid covers skilled care, intermediate care and _____ care

4 The ability of service agencies to understand the world view of clients of different cultures, and adapt practices to ensure their effectiveness (2 wds)

6 The loss of use or availability of funds when cash owed to a facility is not yet in its possession. The value of benefits are sacrificed in order to spend money another way. (2 wds)

8 501 organizations operate primarily for _____ purposes. But, they may regularly engage in business unrelated to exempt purposes (2 wds)

11 Something owned by a facility, which can be converted to cash within twelve months (2 wds)

14 The goal of the Medicaid program changed from expanding services to _____. (2 wds)

16 Workers Compensation insurance is _____ required. It provides for medical/ rehabilitation expenses and/ or cash benefits for illness or injury (regardless of fault)

18 When someone is empowered to act on behalf of a person in case of future incompetence. (4 wds)

20 Under this program, all participating states were to offer comprehensive services to eligible people (the indigent, disabled, blind)

22 True or false: To optimize drug therapy, and minimize errors, there should be separate contracts and payment systems for each, so that the pharmacist who reduces unnecessary drugs is not the same as he who sells the drugs

23 Activities of Daily Living make up ____ percent of the RUG score.

24 The costs associated with salaries, supplies and such, that have been used up through the provision of services

25 In 1935, an Act that guaranteed employee bargaining rights, investigated unfair labor practices, limited employer's freedom to express views on unionization, and defined the rights of workers. The first nationwide labor legislation to favor the growth of trade unions. (aka, National Labor Relations Act)

DOWN

2 This person generates reports on the financial standing of a nursing facility. He or she uses information (such as daily cash transactions) from the bookkeeper, to generate reports.

3 On the federal enforcement grid, this has three levels. It shows the extent of a deficient facility practice on resident outcome (how many residents were affected)

5 An Act, and law that established employer responsibility without regard to fault or negligence for employee's illness or injury that arose out of performance of a job (2 wds)

7 Paid or voluntary staff who investigate nursing home complaints made by residents or family members. They act as resident advocates.

9 An Act that requires any entity that receives five million dollars in annual Medicaid reimbursement to establish written policies for all employees, contractors, and agents, that provide detailed information about the United States False Claims Act and any counterpart state law. (2 wds)

10 A ___ can refuse to release personal or clinical records if required by a duly-appointed state ombudsman.

12 Facilities must notify Medicaid residents when their accounts reach _____ dollars less than the Social Security Income resource limit for one person (2 wds)

13 Liabilities due during the next twelve months. This includes a portion of long-term debt.

15 Type of insurance where an entity assumes its own expenses related to a specific risk of loss by setting aside a determined amount of money periodically, which may be held by a trustee.

17 The accused in criminal cases, the sued in civil cases

19 Medication patches must be labeled when ___.

21 A resident should not have a weight loss that exceeds ___ percent in 30 days

PUZZLE # 37

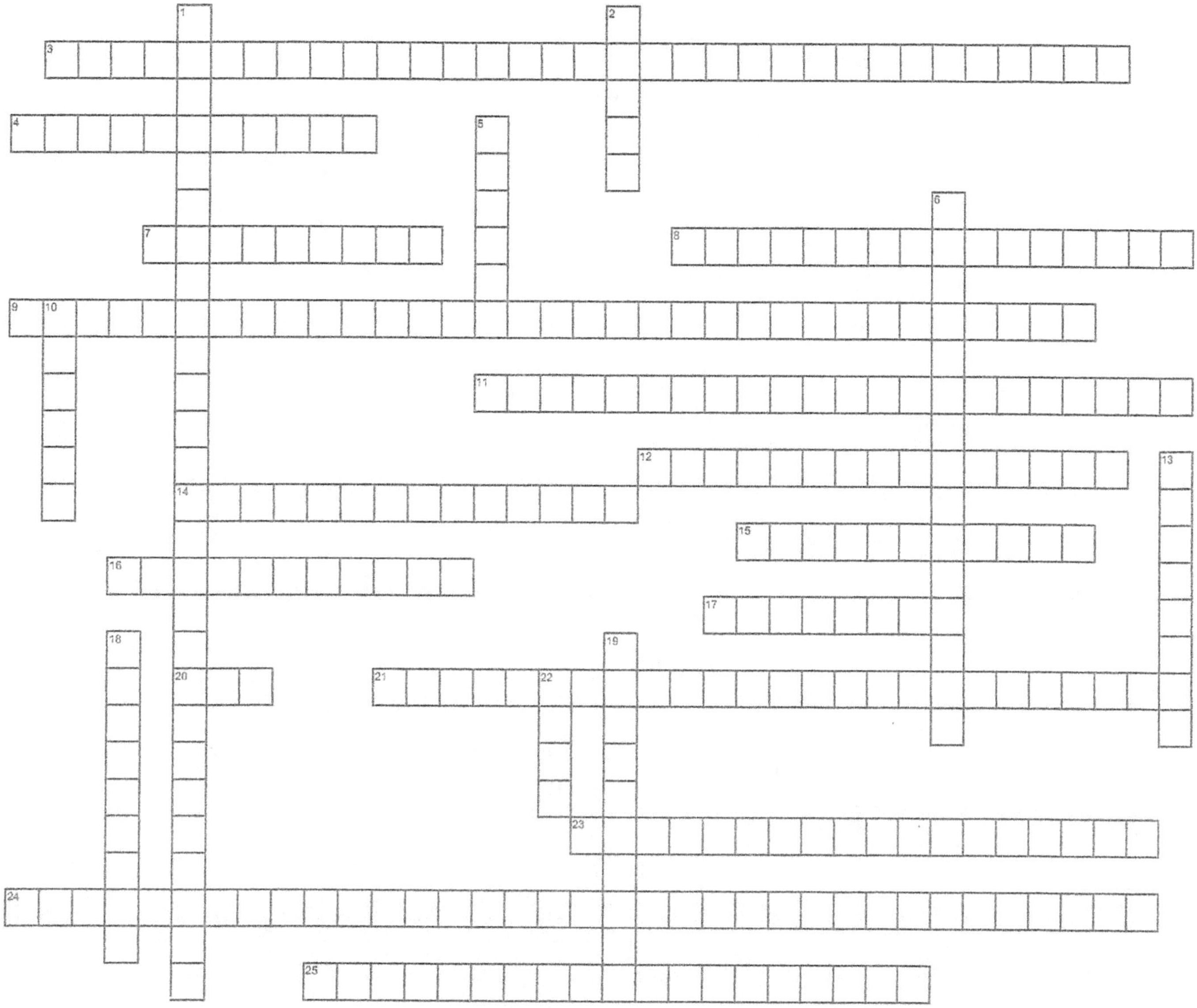

ACROSS

3 C.O.B.R.A. In 1985, this Act provided continued group health coverage for employees and dependents with a qualifying event, such as voluntary or involuntary termination or reduction in hours (unless gross misconduct was involved). (3 wds)
4 Ordinary Power of Attorney ends if a person becomes _____.
7 This type of medication must be double-locked
8 An Act by Congress that gives all states the option of enacting long-term care partnership programs that combine private long-term care insurance with Medicaid coverage. Consumers can pay for long-term care services, and preserve some of their wealth. (2 wds)
9 C.I.O. Major labor group, which merged with the American Federation of Labor in 1955. (4 wds)
11 Examining the facility's goals, resources and internal/ external environments to determine where training is needed (2 wds)
12 Something a facility owns, which cannot be liquidated within one year (such as buildings, property, or equipment). These are fixed, and are recorded at their cost at time of purchase. (2 wds)
14 This records nonrepetitive entries. (2 wds)
15 The person responsible for most personnel functions. This person is delegated authority by the Administrator to make decisions on his or her behalf. This person also has authority to commit facility resources (2 wds)
16 Also known as the "midnight census", this form is completed by nursing staff. (2 wds)
17 Daily volume in long-term care assistance is projected to _____
20 Accumulated Benefit Obligation. The present value of the amount that a facility would owe the pension plan, if all eligible employees retired during that accounting period. (3 initials)
21 C.P.A. This person is licensed to issue an audit opinion on a facility's financial statements (3 wds)
23 The W-5 form is used for this purpose. This form enables advanced payment of income, by having it added to take-home pay during the year. Payments are subtracted from the withheld income tax and FICA taxes (3 wds)
24 I.P.O. An organization that contracts with physicians and provides services to managed care organizations. Physicians are paid (capitation) whether or not patients require care. (3 wds)
25 C.N.A. (3 wds)

DOWN

1 C.I.A. The Office of Inspector General requires that providers adopt specific measures to ensure their integrity regarding fraud and abuse. These measures are detailed in a ______. (3 wds)
2 This type of ratio shows cash and other assets that can be converted to cash right away. Also called the acid-test ratio. The formula is cash plus accounts receivable plus marketable securities, divided by current liabilities
5 Things owned by a facility (this may include trademarks and patents)
6 When the Administrator gives everyone moderate ratings on their evaluations, it is called the error of ____ (2 wds)
10 Medication bottles must be labeled when ____.
13 On the federal enforcement grid, this has four levels. It shows the effect of seriousness of a deficient facility practice on resident outcome (the level of harm)
18 Since 2005, the rules for qualifying for Medicaid have _____
19 When a third party injures the reputation of a victim (can be slander or libel)
22 In 2040, it is projected that the daily volume in long-term care assistance will be ____ times that which was needed in 1980.

PUZZLE # 38

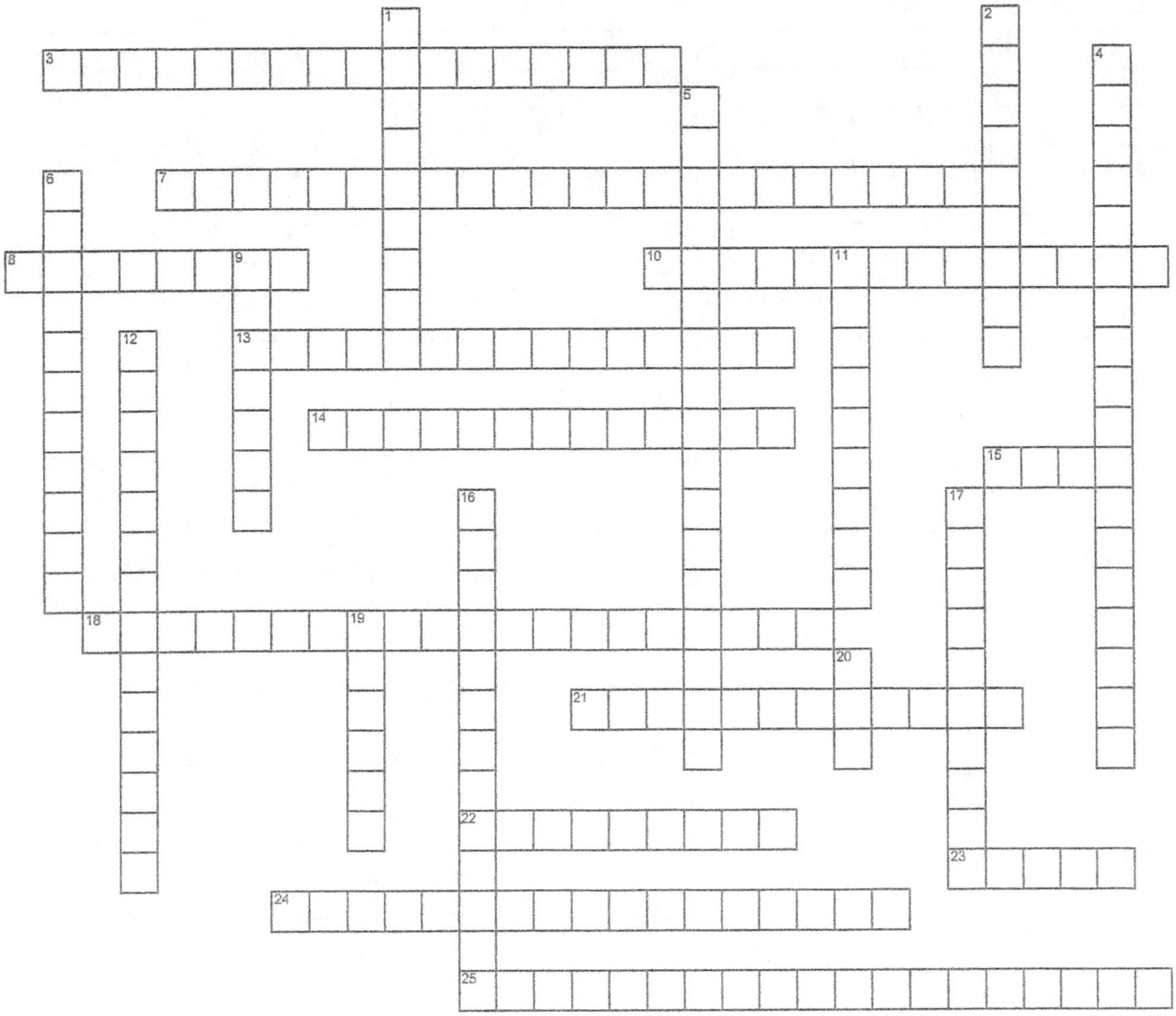

ACROSS

3 This is used to calculate break-even cost in order to analyze the cost effectiveness of such services as physical therapy. Total revenues must equal total expenses (3 wds)

7 An unincorporated association set up to obtain specific goals over a set time period (3 wds)

8 The three parts of a RUG (Resource Utilization Group) are ADL's, therapy, and ________

10 Reasonable anticipation that harm or injury is likely as a result of commission or omission of an act

13 Looking at competitors expansion plans, occupancy levels, and local hospital plans when considering building a new nursing facility. (2 wds)

14 Specific procedures designed to govern the implementation of policies (3 wds)

15 True or false: An employee has two to five days to speak to a supervisor regarding a grievance. The supervisor must then record the grievance.

18 When only one market segment is served. (2 wds)

21 Management universals include planning, organizing, commanding and _____

22 The three sources of law are administrative, common, and ____

23 Type of therapy provided simultaneously to four patients (regardless of payor source) who are performing the same activity

24 Used to plot an organization's direction over three-five years. Includes identifying problems, specifying objectives, creating ideas and alternatives, developing an action plan, gathering and analyzing data, and acting on results (2 wds)

25 When there are as few levels as possible between the Administrator and the rank and file (4 wds)

DOWN

1 The establishment of pay grades and rates by employers to both achieve equity and offer some flexibility to supervisors in setting an employee's wage (2 wds)

2 Promoting and selling products or services. A managerial process that involves analysis, planning, implementation, and control to satisfy consumer and organizational objectives

4 Using audit information to divide potential people served into identifiable groups (2 wds)

5 A projection of the present and future availability of qualified personnel in a number sufficient to meet a facility's needs (2 wds)

6 Criminal negligence, which is the reckless regard of anothers safety. Willful indifference to an injury that could result from an act

9 A fixed amount of money paid periodically by an insurer under the insurance contract terms

11 Management style in which only information that indicates a significant deviation of actual results from planned results are brought to a manager's attention. Management then focuses on really important tactical and strategic tasks

12 The most effective marketing tool is a _______ (3 wds)

16 These provide services during more than one time period. During the course of operation, they lose value as a result of use, wear and tear, or obsolescence. They are purchased for use, not for resale. (2 wds)

17 Recording or reporting the economic condition of various entities

19 Guideline or law that drives processes and procedures. A rule or of a company that ensures consistency and compliance with strategic direction. A guideline under which procedures are developed.

20 Medication Administration Record (3 initials)

PUZZLE # 39

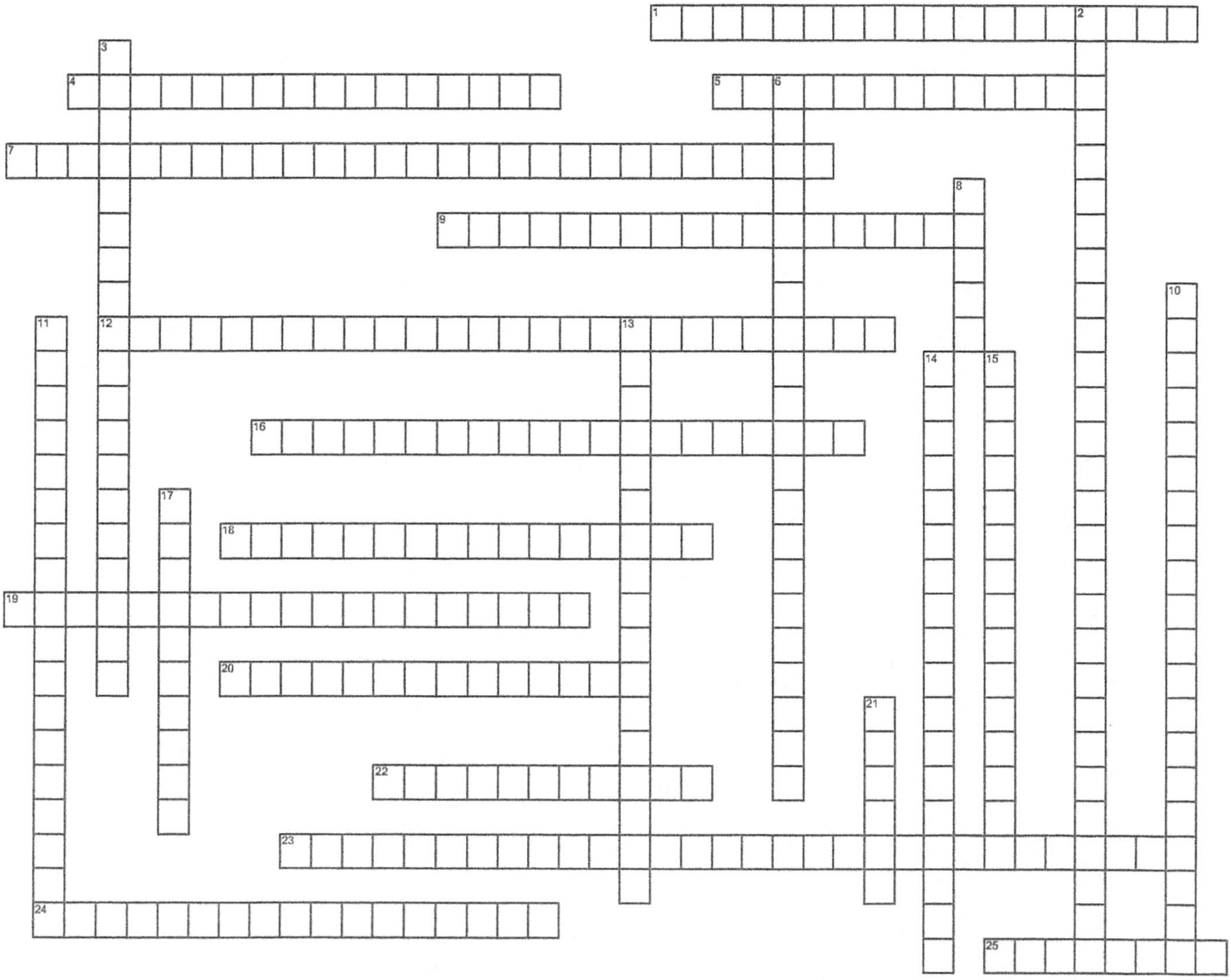

ACROSS

1 Q.I.O. Type of organization that is private, non-profit, and trained to review medical care and help beneficiaries with complaints about care quality, and to implement improvements. CMS contracts with one such organization in every state, and contracts last three years. (2 wds)

4 Q.I. A report that points out potential resident or provider problems. Formulated from MDS information, this is collected on all Medicare and Medicaid patients. It indicates the provider level and resident level status from the MDS. (2 wds)

5 This lists major capital expenditures (such as equipment or buildings), and is planned two years at a time, due to large costs. (2 wds)

7 In 1986, this Act determined who could work in the United States. It stated that all employees hired must be verified as either United States citizens, or otherwise authorized to work in the U.S. Employers must complete Form I-9, which is retained for three years from the hiring date, or one year after an employee is terminated (4 wds)

9 Larger patient census, additional facilities, etc (2 wds)

12 This person has the authority to review all documents to determine compliance with Medicare and Medicaid, and other laws. He or she monitors documentation and facility programs that are relevant to Medicare and Medicaid's conditions of participation. The OIG mandates that each facility has one. (3 wds)

16 A.P.R. Measures the true cost of credit (3 wds)

18 A concept that treats each business as a separate reporting entity from the personal affairs of those who manage or own it (2 wds)

19 Identifies how investors should choose common stocks for their portfolio, under a given set of assumptions (3 wds)

20 Publicly reported information (through CMS) to help consumers assess quality of care. There are two categories: conditions relevant to long-term care residents, and conditions relevant to short-stay residents. (2 wds)

22 Quality of life and quantity of life are ___

23 O.B.R.A. This provided the statutory authority for MDS's, and required skilled nursing facilities and nursing facilities to do initial and periodic assessments of all residents. Also, it included configuring inputs (such as the amount of floor space per resident). Finally, it promoted quality of life, rights, choices and personal care. (4 wds)

24 A range of activities that the court considers the legal responsibility of the employer. (In other words, any act done as part of one's duties) (3 wds)

25 Thirty-year treasury bonds that mature beyond ten years (2 wds)

DOWN

2 Designed to reduce or eliminate the need for excessive inventories. Determines how much material to purchase, in order to meet a facility's needs (3 wds)

3 Associating two or more companies (2 wds)

6 Also called Malpractice Insurance, type of insurance that protects against claims of negligence (2 wds)

8 Number of management layers in tasks in a 120+ bed facility

10 Type of insurance that covers loss of income from a reduction or stoppage of business activity caused by fire or other insured peril (2 wds)

11 A.D.C. (3 wds)

13 C.O.N. Half of all states have done away with these, and since 1986 they have been at the state level. They are issued when additional nursing facilities are warranted (3 wds)

14 In 1990, this Act states that healthcare facilities must report accidents or incidents related to a medical device, that caused or contributed to injury, illness or death to a resident or employee. Reports must be filed with the FDA within ten days if a death occurred. Reports must be made with the manufacturer if serious illness or injury occur. All records are maintained for two years from the filing date. (3 wds)

15 S.D.S. (used to be M.S.D.S.) (3 wds)

17 The grouping of activities and the people who will carry them out. Assigning roles. Delegating authority.

21 For quality indicators, the broad areas of care the represent the common conditions and important aspects of care and life to nursing facility residents. Each one is represented by one or more quality indicators

PUZZLE # 40

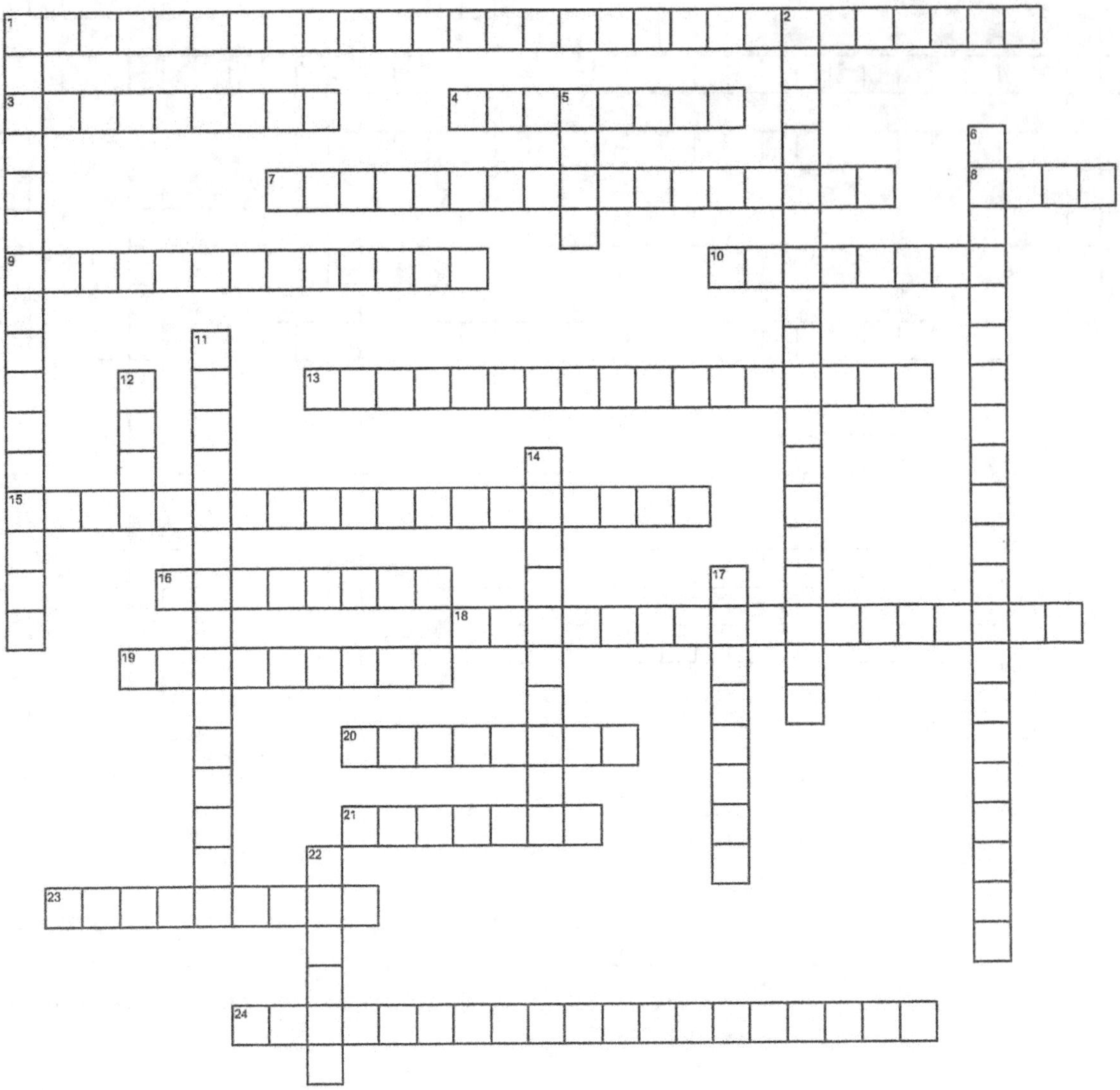

ACROSS

1 This prolongs the shelf life of fresh or minimally processed foods, and must be inspected for time and/or temperature abuse (3 wds)

3 The Cumulative Effect of a Change in Accounting Principle describes the effect of _____ from one accounting principle to another (in regards to the income statement)

4 To deliver a drug to a resident

7 A devise which prevents or restricts resident movement. (2 wds)

8 Resource Utilization Groups. A collection of nursing facility resident classification systems used in a variety of case mix indexed reimbursement systems. (4 initials)

9 This is used for Medicare Prospective Payment System assessments. It encompasses a specific time frame and look-back period to review services used. (2 wds)

10 Assistance given to a subordinate

13 A psychoactive drug used for discipline of a resident, rather than medical treatment (2 wds)

15 Altering the consistency of food for a resident, to assist with chewing or swallowing. (2 wds)

16 Favoritism of family members in hiring practices

18 S.P. This person is licensed,certified or registered by state statute (2 wds)

19 The granting of a license to a provider who meets state requirements for operation

20 These assets have future economic benefits that are expected to last for years (2 wds)

21 Type of corporation that exists without authorization by law. Three conditions must be met: A statute exists under which it can be categorized, it behaves and functions like a corporation, and it assumes some corporation privileges (2 wds)

23 Type of resident stay, where admission to discharge is completed in under fourteen days (2 wds)

24 This Act states that an employer must tell applicants in a credit report will be requested. If a candidate is rejected due to poor credit, he or she must be told so, and must be given the name and address of a reporting credit agency. (3 wds)

DOWN

1 The deliberate misplacement, exploitation or wrongful use of a resident's belongings or money, without the resident's consent

2 C.P.M. (3 wds)

5 Program Evaluation and Review Technique. Control tools which show the relationship among the activities which make up a project (4 initials)

6 Use of a specified number of verbal warnings, then more stern written warnings for each offense of the same rule before suspending or firing an employee (2 wds)

11 When someone has the necessary information to make a healthcare decision. (2 wds)

12 How a person walks

14 When a supervisor values one particular job behavior over others, and bases his or her opinion of other traits on the absence or presence of that one behavior (2 wds)

17 A compilation of facility policies that relate to work conditions. Often considered binding in a court of law

22 Revenue remaining after expenses are paid.

PUZZLE # 41

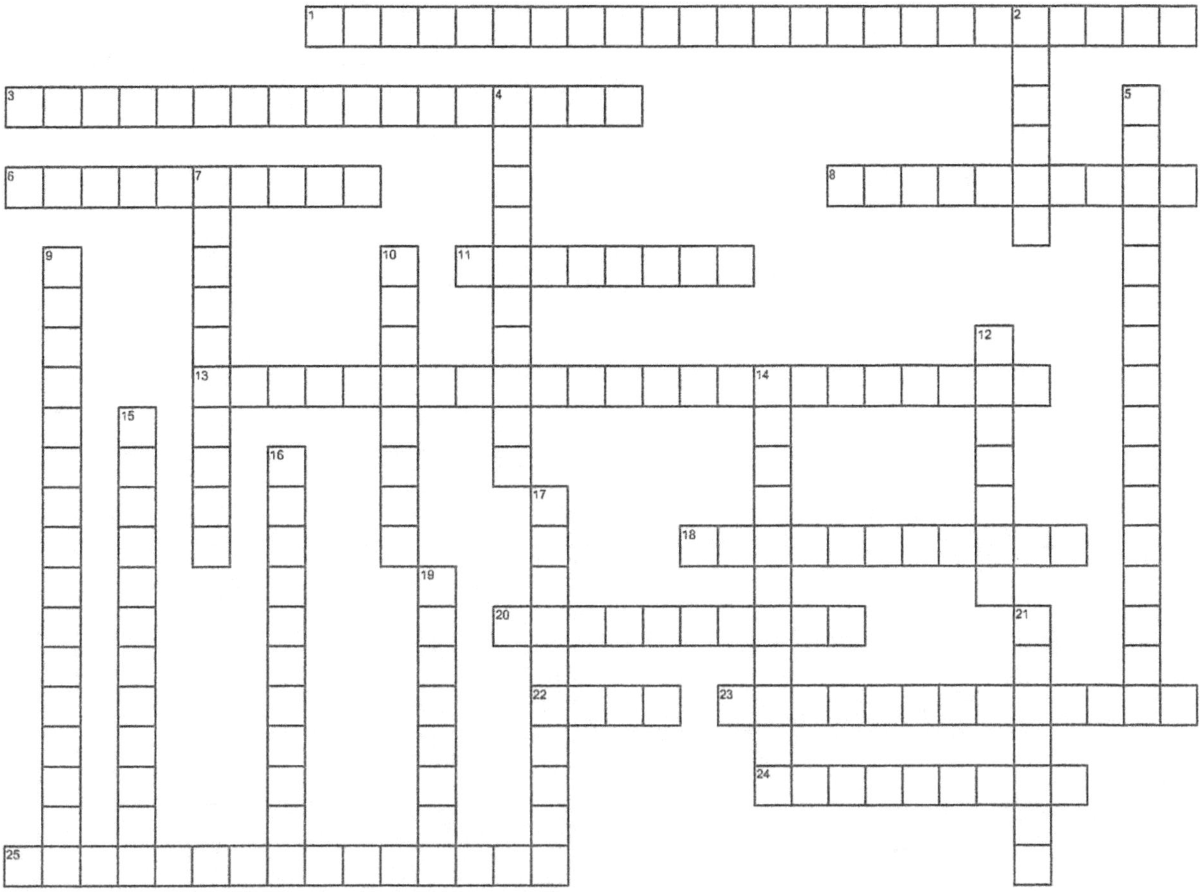

ACROSS

1 This system must supply enough power to light all entrances and exits, all equipment to maintain fire detection, all alarm and extinguishing systems, and life-supporting systems (3 wds)
3 A major decline or improvement in a resident's condition, which usually requires intervention from staff, and usually impacts more than one area of a resident's health. (2 wds)
6 Able to walk, with or without difficulty or help
8 This person is in charge of finding a defendant guilty
11 Type of program provided to residents who cannot plan their own activity pursuits, or to residents who need specialized or extended programs to enhance their overall daily routine (3 wds)
13 A.P.S. Part of the Adult and Family Services Division, they investigate reports of abuse, neglect, and exploitation of those age 60 and over, and incapacitated adults age 18+. They provide health, housing, social and legal services (3 wds)
18 A loss of the body's normal water content.
20 Type of intervention that does not rely on medication. May include changing a resident's environment to promote change in behavior
22 Skin ulcers fall under ___ categories
23 A financial statement that lists an excess of revenues over expenses of operation, interest income and owners equity (contributions to a facility). (3 wds)
24 The formation of a _____ happens when the body weight exerts unusual pressure on internal soft tissues (2 wds)
25 L.B.O. When controlling interest in a company is purchased, using debt. Collaterized by target company's assets to fund most or all of the purchase price. (3 wds)

DOWN

2 A generalized statement of intention
4 The direct application of a vaccine or a prescribed drug or device, whether by injection, ingestion or any other means, to a resident
5 Type of culture where the management makes the decisions, and residents are expected to follow existing routines. (2 wds)
7 The inhalation of a foreign object, into the lungs.
9 This ratio measures the number of times a company can make its interest payment with its earnings, before interest and taxes. The formula is EBITDA divided by interest expense. (2 wds)
10 Type of insurance that covers physical damage to a building and its contents
12 Compensation, other than cash wages. (may include vacation time, paid health insurance)
14 Federal regulations that define safe practices that, when adhered to, will not be considered violations to the federal anti-kickback. (2 wds)
15 Lacking voluntary control over the bladder or bowel
16 The nurse in charge of a specific part of a facility during a specific shift (2 wds)
17 An undesirable effect of a medication. (2 wds)
19 Any non-routine endeavor which a resident participates in, that is meant to enhance his or her sense of well-being and to promote or enhance physical, cognitive and emotional health.
21 Over _____ thousand people/ places are included on a list of Excluded Individuals/ Entities, through the OIG, that are prohibited from having Medicare or Medicaid, or other federal healthcare programs.

PUZZLE # 42

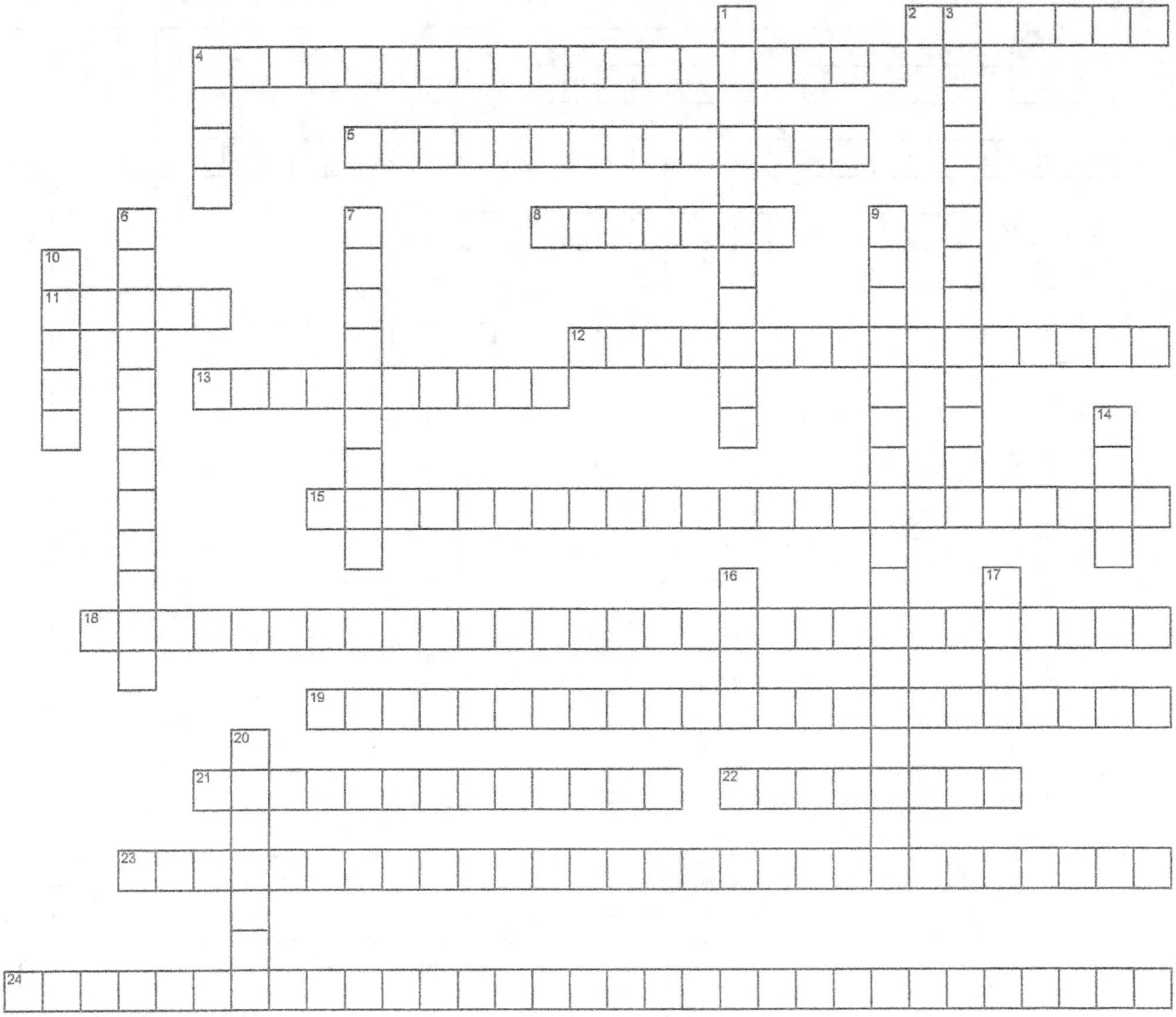

1
2
3
4
5
6
7
8
9
10
11
12
13
14
15
16
17
18
19
20
21
22
23
24

ACROSS

2 Bonds are rated by ___ credit rating agencies

4 A program that reduces chemical-related occupational illness and/or injury. (2 wds)

5 This concept relates to how all financial information must be shown in a facility's financial records (2 wds)

8 This concept relates to all aspects of how things in a skilled nursing facility/ nursing facility are going

11 Health Insurance Prospective Payment System code. A five-position code for billing Part A covered days to the Part A Medicare Administration Contractor (MAC) (5 initials)

12 Systematic activites performed to determine the extent to which clinical practice meets specified standards and values with regard to appropriate services and their duration, appropriate facilities and resources used, and adequate and clinical soundness of given care. (2 wds)

13 Buildings with life support systems must have emergency lighting equipment supplied by the life safety branch of the _____ system

15 Creating awareness among potential customers regarding services, assisting them in deciding, and assuring that they are satisfied with the quality of services (2 wds)

18 Type of insurance that covers statutory liability regarding bodily injury, sickness, death from an accident arising from the maintenance or use of a facility's property, or accidents caused by employees while working (3 wds)

19 The two items necessary to ensure that a claim reflects assessment information are the HIPPS code (Health Insurance Prospective Payment System) and this (3 wds)

21 Patient room doors must be made of _____ (3 wds)

22 Approximately what percent of Medicaid recipients have five or more chronic conditions?

23 A process that utilizes the team approach to improving an organization (3 wds)

24 F.I.C.A. An employee's contribution to the Social Security fund. (4 wds) (4 wds)

DOWN

1 In 1986, this Act authorized damages up to three times the amount of fraud and civil monetary penalties of $11,000.00 per false claim. (2 wds)

3 One part of the operational budget. Projects monthly income for next year. (2 wds)

4 Hours per patient day. An OBRA regulation. (4 initials)

6 A means of allocating the cost of a long-term asset over its useful life.

7 This form of assessment is done when a Medicare Part A patient discharges from a facility on or before day #8, and that resident completed one-four days of therapy, which began at some point during the last four days (2 wds)

9 A staff member who assists line managers in record-keeping, recruitment, selection, and the training and retraining of employees. This person is responsible for human resource functions, and is usually a full-time team member in facilities with 100 or more beds (2 wds)

10 In 2006, less than ___% of nursing facilities received deficiencies in resident rights

14 Each patient room must have either an outside window, or a ___. (If a window, it does not have to actually work)

16 True or false: Using several depreciation schedules for one piece of equipment is acceptable

17 Meals on Wheels must deliver at least ___ times a week. (they must also provide 1/3 of the daily nutritional requirements for a resident)

20 Asking if actual output is up to standards, and if not, taking corrective actions

PUZZLE # 43

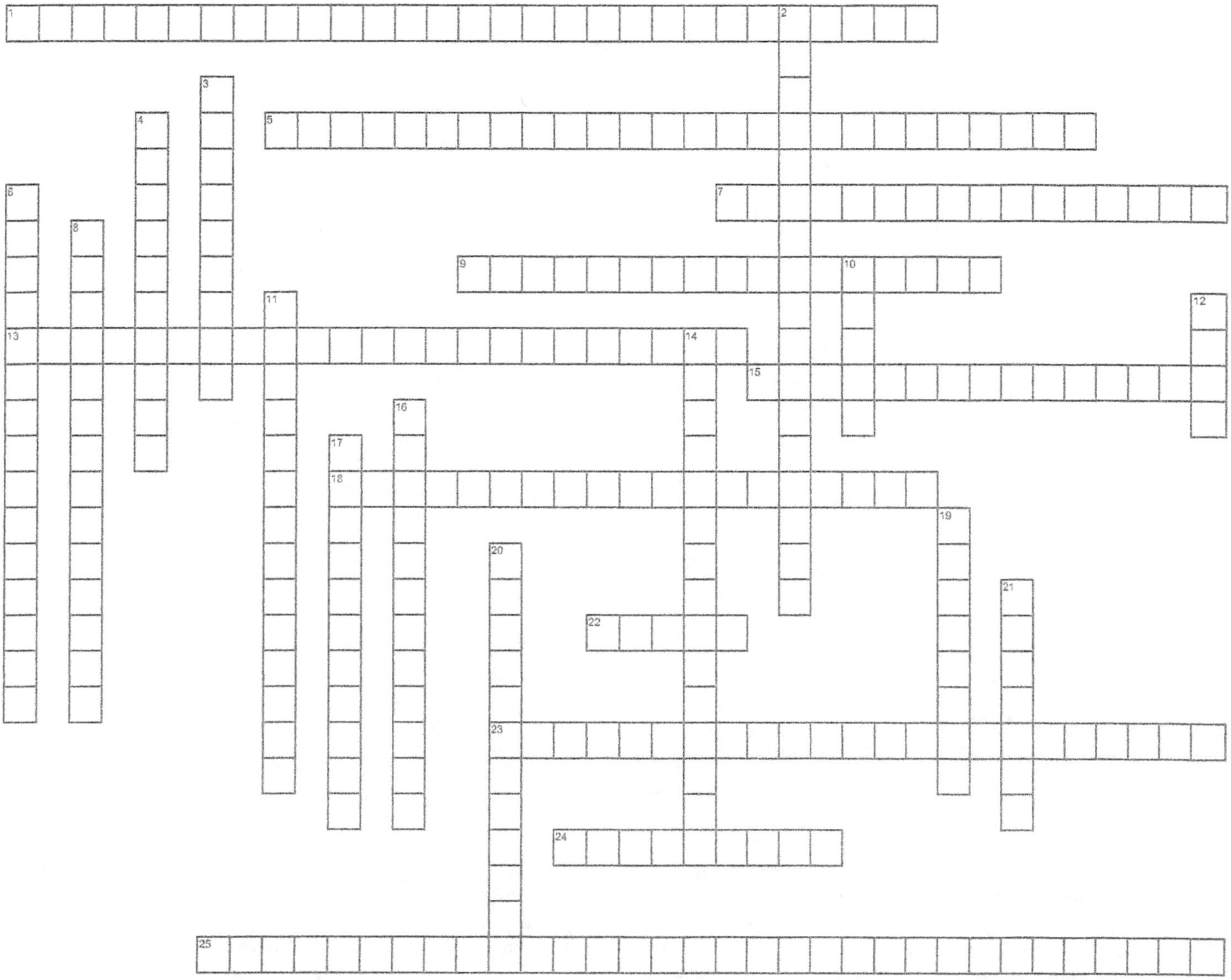

ACROSS

1 PPO. A form of managed care organization. More flexible than an HMO; can see a specialist without first seeing primary care; high deductible for convenience (3 wds)

5 In the 1920's, this describes when private citizens gathered to discuss health legislation (4 wds)

7 Type of partnership that limits a partner's liability to the general contractual debts, the partner's individual malpractice, and wrongful acts of people acting under a partner's direct supervision (2 wds)

9 Selecting a target market, choosing a competitive position, and developing an effective marketing mix to reach and serve identified customers (2 wds)

13 Working in several product markets (2 wds)

15 Also known as Return on Services Rendered, this shows the percentage of net income generated by each service-billed dollar in for-profit facilities. The formula is net income after tax, divided by sales (3 wds)

18 What type of medication must be separately locked from other medications? (2 wds)

22 These costs do not relate to changes in volume. They do not change when volume changes. (examples: salary, depreciation, rent)

23 This person is in charge of all clinical and operational aspects of the dietary department (3 wds)

24 Approximately what percent of Medicaid recipients are female? (2 wds)

25 E.R.I.S.A. In 1975, this Act set minimum funding for pension funds, required certification every three years, and required vesting of employee's equity in the pension fund. (4 wds)

DOWN

2 The federal government's review of hiring practices (recruiting, advertising, data retained on applicants) to ensure conformity of the 1964 Civil Rights Act and amendments. (2 wds)

3 In patient rooms, windows must be _____ inches from the floor (in other words, sill height) (2 wds)

4 Another term for "physician's orders" (2 wds)

6 Bonds with a low risk of default are ____ (2 wds)

8 Taking steps to assure that goals are accomplished and that each job is well done (2 wds)

10 The American Institute of Certified Public Accountants. A national organization of CPA's, who develop standards for members, and offer advice to the S.E.C. (5 initials)

11 for CHSRA quality indicators, a way to rank providers on how they compare with each other on each indicator. The higher the rank, the better (2 wds)

12 Bonds with a high risk of default are called ___ bonds (also known as high-yield bonds)

14 In laundry, wash should be done at ___ degrees or higher, for twenty-five minutes (3 wds)

16 When an organization seeks to improve its business practices by comparing them with the best practices of other organizations.

17 What class of medication is not permitted in a facility? (2 wds)

19 Practices that lead to exceptional performance

20 A long-term rental agreement between the lessor and lessee that runs for the entire useful life of an asset (2 wds)

21 The local job market, prevailing wage rates, cost-of-living increases, collective bargaining, individual bargaining, and the value of a job all contribute toward determining the _____ (2 wds)

PUZZLE # 44

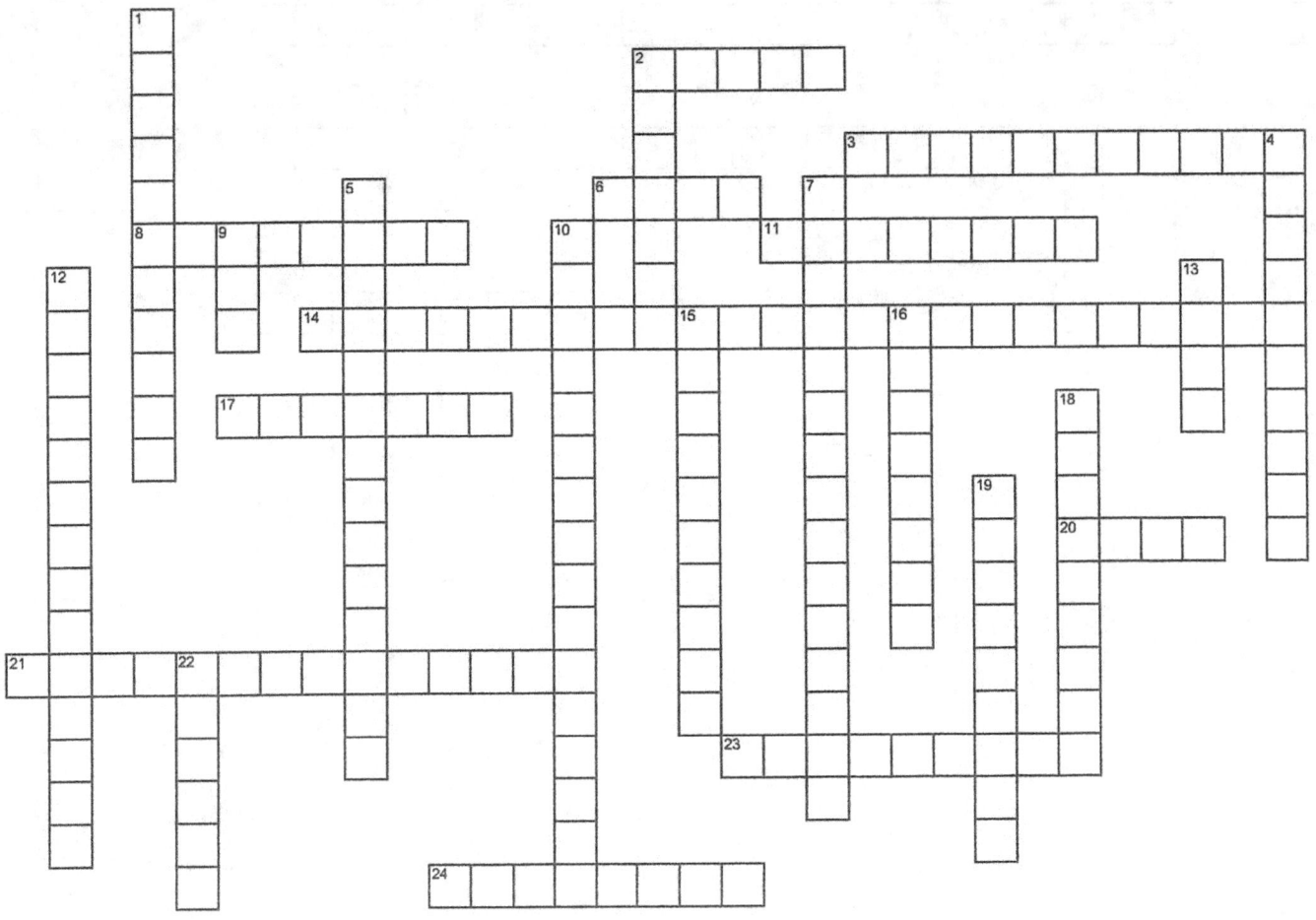
1
2
3
4
5
6
7
8
9
10
11
12
13
14
15
16
17
18
19
20
21
22
23
24

ACROSS

2 The approximate percent of Medicaid recipients age 65 or older.

3 The class of medication that must be accounted for on every shift (2 wds)

6 A substance used in the diagnosis, cure, mitigation, treatment or prevention of a health condition.

8 Set of laws that prohibit the practice of self-referral by physicians (2 wds)

11 Type of insurance that covers the aged, the blind, the medically needy, and the permanently and totally disabled.

14 This Act requires facilities to recognize a patient's living will or Power of Attorney as their Advanced Directive (3 wds)

17 This mean "effectiveness". It is the status of care provided to a resident. It impacts the level of satisfaction to a customer, and determines the facility's quality. If it is deficient, surveyor's will look at the processes which the facility uses to provide care.

20 True or False: In dietary, the refrigerator and freezer must have thermometers, temperatures must be monitored and recorded, and adequate space must be provided.

21 This assigns each patient to a caseworker, who helps design a care plan from different agencies (2 wds)

23 Three types of long-term care are skilled, intermediate, and ___.

24 An advance gained by using debt financing to create asset appreciation

DOWN

1 Three types of business combinations are statutory merger, statutory consolidation and ___.

2 The Nation's highest court. The only Federal court created by the Constitution.

4 The first step toward implementing a plan; a managerial behavior

5 This Act requires prospective payments for care given, drastically reducing cash flow to home health agencies. It also mandates the use of a prospective payment system for SNF's and home health care. It gave permission to states to allow mandated enrollment in a MCO as a condition of getting Medicaid assistance (2 wds)

7 That which is incurred in one account period, but benefits future periods (2 wds)

9 Assessment Reference Date (3 initials)

10 Type of facility that is now known as a nursing facility (NF) (since 1990) (2 wds)

12 The process of explaining and correcting any discrepancies between a bank statement balance and depositor's record of cash balance

13 Minimum width for wheelchairs to pass is __ feet.

15 Automatic or power-assisted doors must be slow-opening and ____. They must not open back-to-back faster than three seconds, nor with a force exceeding fifteen pounds.

16 Capital cost items are either categorized as capitalized or ____.

18 Type of care that includes providing assistance with ADL's. No doctor's orders are required, and this type of care can be provided by non-professionals. (NOT covered by Medigap or Medicare insurances)

19 Managerial success includes ___ for the future

22 Someone who advises another, over a period of time

PUZZLE # 45

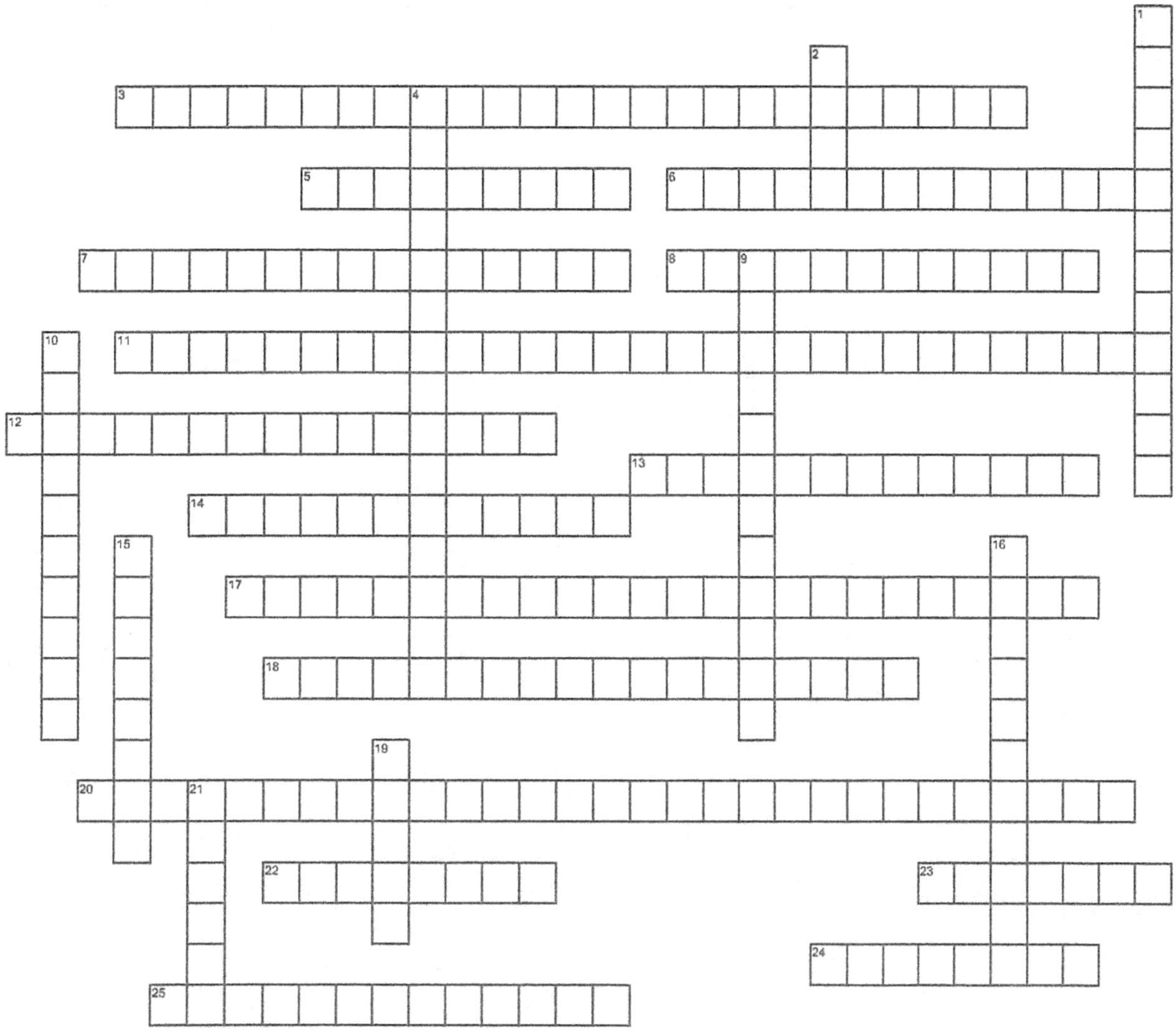

1
2
3
4
5
6
7
8
9
10
11
12
13
14
15
16
17
18
19
20
21
22
23
24
25

ACROSS

3 P.I.P. Quality indicator information system for long-term care, developed by CHSRA, that utilizes MDS assessment data. (3 wds)

5 The ARD (assessment reference date) for an assessment is always day of ____

6 This pricing is based on buyer's perception of the value of a product or service, rather than seller's cost. (good reputation= higher rates) (2 wds)

7 This ratio indicates profitability relative to total revenue. It is shown on a consolidated basis as well as per business unit. The formula is net operating income divided by total revenue. (2 wds)

8 Type of negligence where the victim is partly responsible. All recovery by the victim is barred. (example: Use of a product in ways it was not intended to be used)

11 Q.A.A. Type of committee that identifies quality deficiencies that require action, and develops plans of action to correct them. They also monitor the effects of those corrections. (Every facility must have a Q.A.A. committee, which meets quarterly) (4 wds)

12 Short-term securities (2-270 days) issued by corporation's banks to raise short-term working capital (unsecured debt). (2 wds)

13 A summary of all debts and credits contained in the journals for a time period (2 wds)

14 Type of depreciation, where most of the expense is in the early years of the asset's life. This enables the owner to receive tax and/or reimbursement benefits more quickly

17 O.I.G. They specifically target four billing practices (claims for services not provided, claims for beneficiaries not home-bound, claims for visits not made, and claims for visits not authorized by physician). They have a nationwide program of audits, inspections and investigations. (3 wds)

18 A legal corporation of two or more partners, with limited liability and joint management by partners. Profits and losses are shared. (3 wds)

20 H.M.O. A form of managed care. Low monthly premiums, no deductible, low co-pays, allows preventive services, provides incentives to prevent unnecessary care. A list of acceptable providers must be chosen from. Primary care treatment is expected, before emergency room visits or specialist appointments (3 wds)

22 The number of nursing facility residents on psychoactive drugs in 2006 was ____ percent (2 wds)

23 This type of nursing facility is Medicare certified, and is considered the highest level of care

24 These costs are not directly associated with a revenue center, yet they support the functions of resident care centers. (also known as support service costs) (examples: payroll, dietary, laundry)

25 Who must provide a written copy of the evacuation plan?

DOWN

1 Style of management that establishes an internally equitable and externally competitive philosophy and practice for paying employees. A means to attract and retain employees. Through this style, management assists department heads and the payroll office in administering salary and other benefits offered by a facility.

2 True or false: Employee's are permitted to have a portable heater in their lounge, as long as it does not exceed 212 degrees Fahrenheit

4 Which financial document shows the net income of a facility? (in other words, the "bottom line") (2 wds)

9 Revenues that include internal income, borrowed funds, and charitable donations

10 The product lines and items that a facility offers. The products that an Administrator wants to serve in a SNF/ NF. (2 wds)

15 A discharge assessment must be sent to CMS within ___ days of discharge

16 A set of services within the "product mix" that are closely related (due to functional similarity) (2 wds)

19 The number of chair-bound residents in nursing facilities in 2006 was just over ____ percent

21 Adequate staff must be maintained, and staff must have access to keys whenever a door is ___

PUZZLE # 46

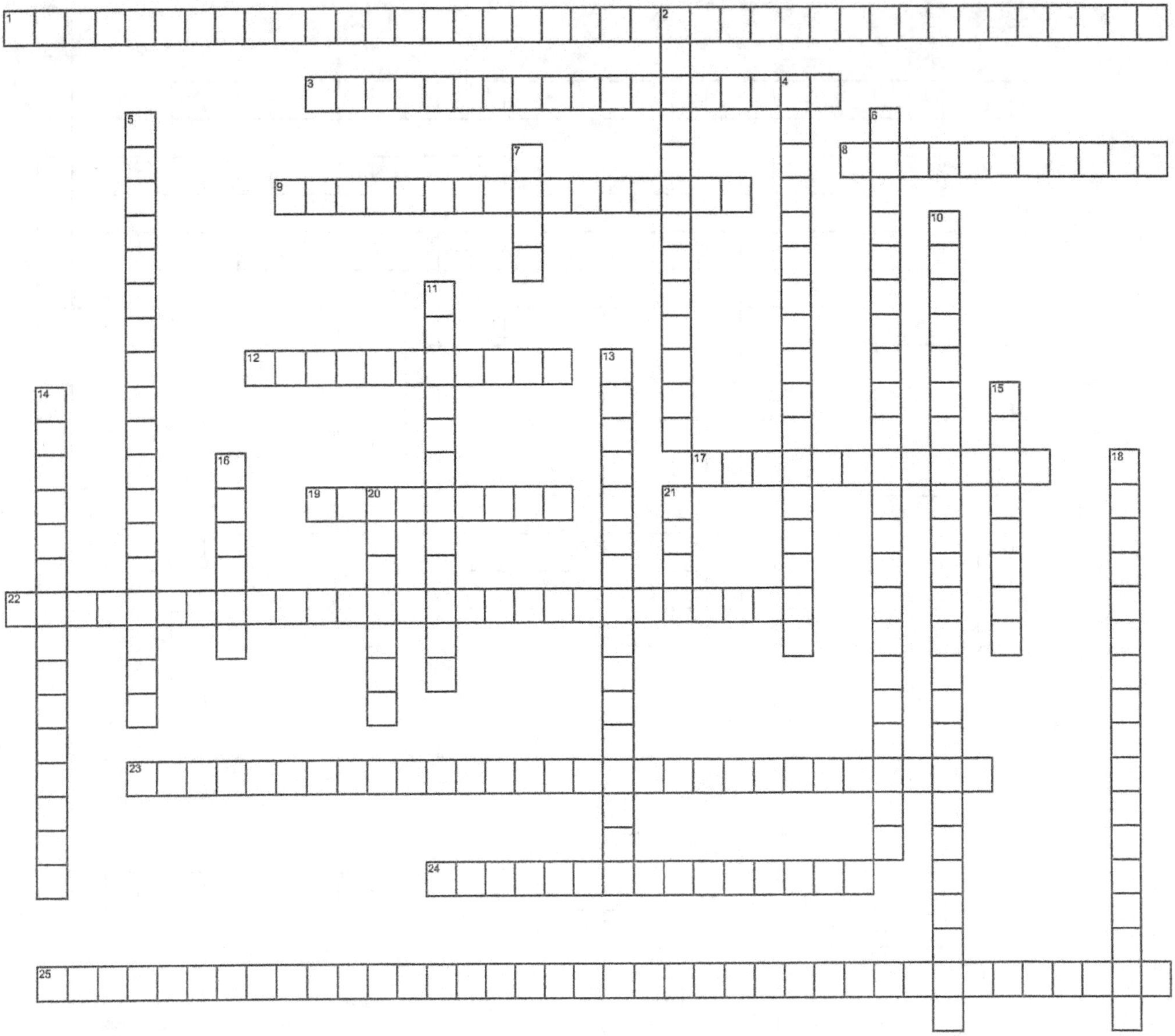

ACROSS

1 A CMS program that compiles information about nursing home residents on eight situations/ conditions called quality measures, and makes that information available to consumers (5 wds)

3 C.P.I. Government-defined measure of the cost of living compared to a base point, which is designated at 100%. (3 wds)

8 When one assessment satisfies both OBRA and Medicare requirements, it may be used as an assessment ____

9 When a manufacturer, seller or supplier to a buyer or third party is accountable for injuries sustained due to a defect in a product. (2 wds)

12 An S Corporation pays federal taxes as a _____. (In order to have "S" status, it must be a domestic corporation, it must not own 80% of another corporation's stock, it must have no more than 35 shareholders, and it must not have any non-resident (alien) shareholders.

17 Type of management that sets specific goals with a time frame for achievement and performance feedback. Lower level employees participate, recommendations move upward, and the final selection of goals are made by upper management. (2 wds)

19 Common responses to a new suggestion. Resistance.

22 Program that maintains clinical records, compliant with accepted professional standards and practices. (Records are kept as long as the state requires, or five years from discharge date) (3 wds)

23 Stating training goals in terms of behaviors that can be learned and observed by supervisors or others. (example: the ability to demonstrate proper procedures for preventing pressure ulcers) (3 wds)

24 To assist the federal government's tracking of beneficiaries' benefit periods, Medicare SNF's must submit "no pay" and ________ claims at specific times, even when no benefits may be payable (2 wds)

25 F.M.C.S. A federal agency that prohibits giving tenure or wage increases to discourage unionization. (5 wds)

DOWN

2 Hot food must be stored at _____ degrees (3 wds)

4 This Act contains statutes (in various states) that set forth the extent to which employers are liable in regard to employees (2 wds)

5 The formula costs in a month, divided by total patient days in a month is _____ (4 wds)

6 The process that consumers go through before, during and after a decision to purchase a product or service (3 wds)

7 The maximum permitted pounds of pressure to operate doors or windows is ___

10 Maximizing the communication and facility acceptance by non-unionized employees in the hope that they will feel no need to form a union to achieve their work goals (3 wds)

11 The most common type of depreciation, where costs are allocated uniformly over an asset's estimated life. (historical cost divided by useful life= annual depreciation). Most third-party payers require this type of depreciation (2 wds)

13 In 1890, an Act that was a landmark federal statute on the United States competition law. Prohibited anti-competitive behaviors, and limited cartels and monopolies (2 wds)

14 Someone who is temporarily employed by another (2 wds)

15 Hot food must leave the kitchen at ___ degrees (2 wds)

16 Who stated that there are four steps quality control and improvement? (plan, do, study and act)

18 This act defines Medicare and Medicaid. The original Act enacted the program, authorized taxes and established administrative mechanisms. (3 wds)

20 Deming stated that evaluation by performance, merit ratings, and annual reviews of performance destroy teamwork and nuture _____

21 Data Assessment and Verification Program. A program administered by CMS, designed to ensure accuracy of MDS data (accomplished through data analysis, off-site review, on-site review and provider education) (4 initials)

PUZZLE # 47

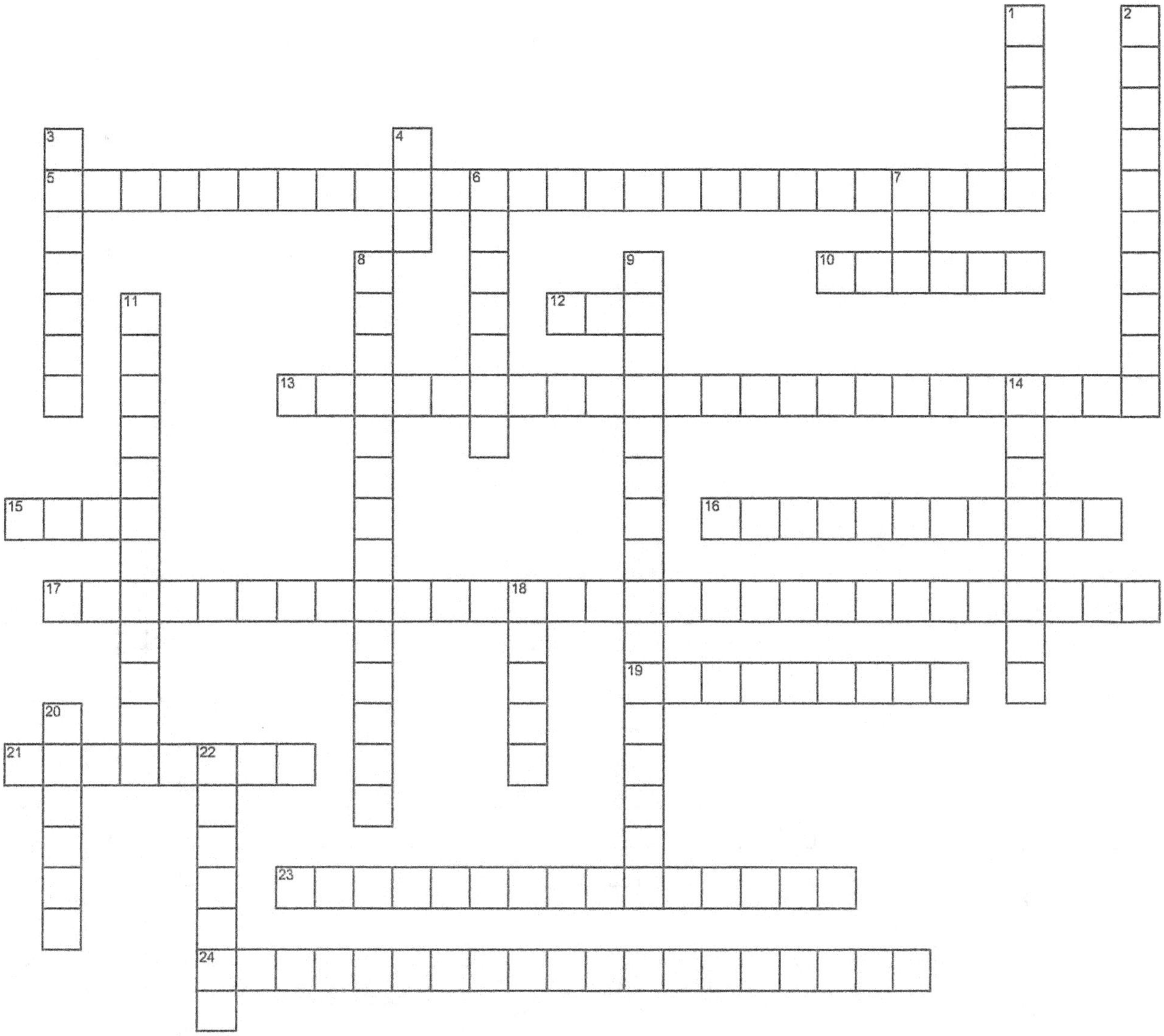

ACROSS

5 This authorization form, signed by a resident or legal representative, requests that his or her medical record information is released to a third party. (4 wds)

10 All cash must be handled by at least two employees, and both employees must be _____

12 Every patient treatment floor must have at least ___ smoke compartments. (Every floor with 50 or more occupants, regardless of purpose/ use, must have the same amount of smoke compartments)

13 An accounting concept of an excess amount over par value that shareholders pay for company stock. Usually treated as a donation. (4 wds)

15 The decision-making process is more complicated than the simple establishment of lower, middle, and upper levels of management

16 Labs and _______ make a big difference in cost of care, for a resident

17 This Act protects against ageism. Today, mandatory retirement is illegal. (4 wds)

19 A ____ must approve and confirm the use of physical restraints within one hour of use. (The legal representative or family member associated with the resident must be notified within the first twelve hours)

21 Type of therapy for musculoskeletal disorders

23 Handrails and grab bars must have a stress point of ____ pounds or greater (3 wds)

24 O.T. Focuses on the use of upper extremities to perform various tasks. Evaluates and treats functional impairments in Activities of Daily Living. Evaluates independent living environment when a patient is scheduled for discharge. (2 wds)

DOWN

1 The Change Of Therapy window is ___ days

2 These objectives are measured by observing if staff exhibit the behaviors sought as the objective of their training, when doing their duties (1 wds)

3 Many food allergies are caused by ____

4 Comprehensive Health Planning (Act): In 1966, this Act was the federal government's first health planning law. It mandated that consumers must make up 51% of the Board and have active voices in program planning. (3 initials)

6 Who said that organizations tend to treat employees as immature, which results in department heads who conform, are defensive, produce detailed stuff on trivial problems, and give invalid information.

7 A resident in physical restraints should be provided motion, exercise, elimination for ___ minutes every hour.

8 A statement of tasks to be done based on the job analysis. Usually includes a list of duties and responsibilities of the position, in order of their importance. (Information about a job, and a list of its duties) (2 wds)

9 This ratio shows the average lag time of account receivables. (2 wds)

11 This type of journal records all cash received for services provided (2 wds)

14 Type of communication that is within and between groups in a facility (examples: one nurse to another, dietary aid to dietary aid

18 Summarizing account receivables (unpaid balances) in terms of how old they are. One step in the collection process, in reporting on the balance sheet a deduction from account receivables for estimated bad debt, and in making write-off decisions

20 _____ should be signed by two employees

22 The corrective action taken after the evaluation of outputs by the organizations decision makers. (If outputs do not meet expectations, these actions bring outputs in line with those that were planned)

PUZZLE # 48

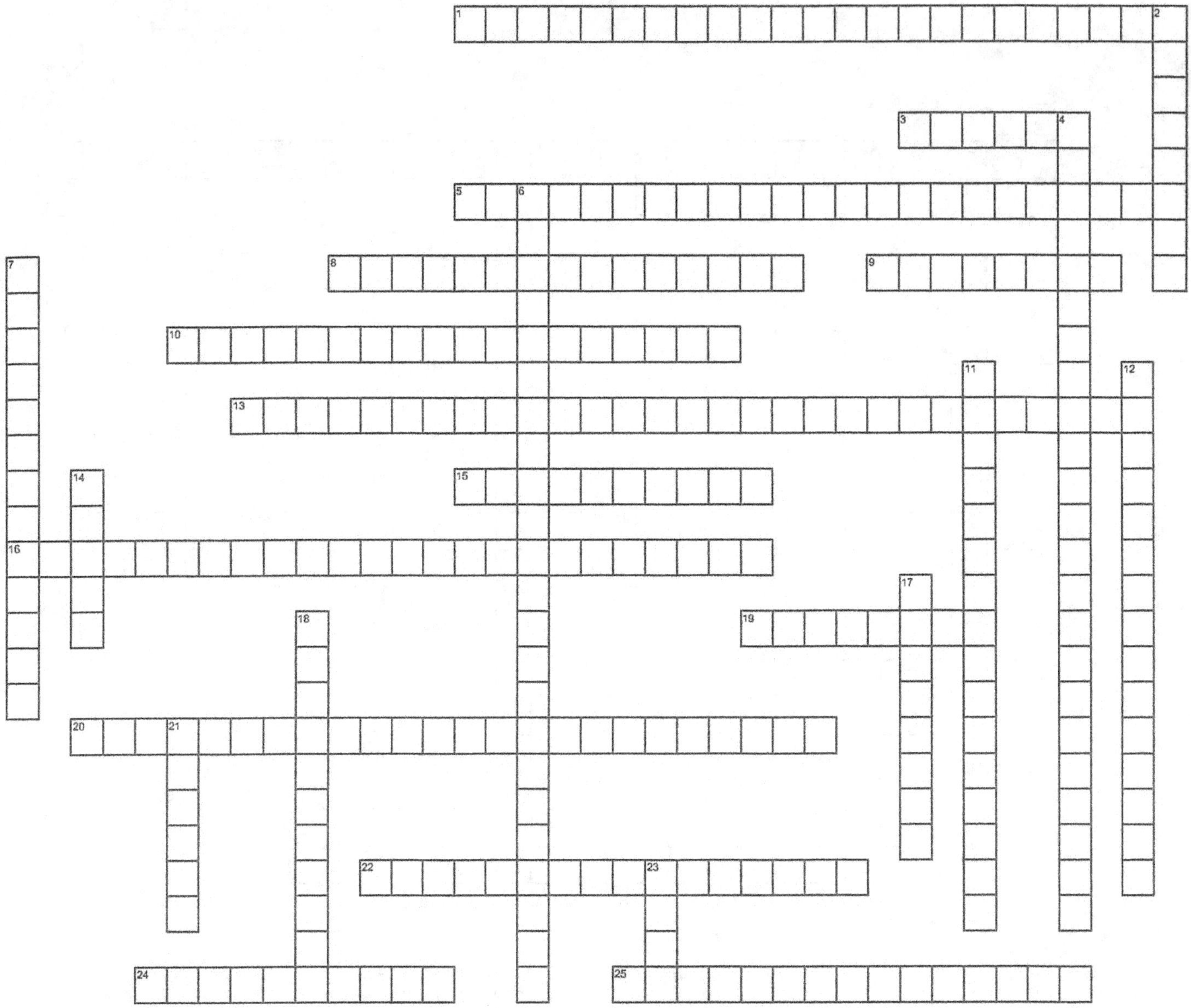

ACROSS

1 An optional employee benefit where employees can set aside a set amount of funds for future medical services. (Funds that are not used, and not carried into the next fiscal year) (3 wds)

3 Type of communication which may be downward or upward

5 A revision in an accounting forecast/ assumption about a facility's expected or experienced performance (4 wds)

8 Using false or fraudulent pretences, representations or promises to obtain property from more than one person (3 wds)

9 Details about the infection control program, such as the size of the committee, the scope of work, the reporting requirements are up to the ____

10 A set-aside portion of retained earnings (equal to depreciation expense) in a separate account, designated to be used only for the purchase of replacement capital assets (2 wds)

13 A.H.C.A. The nation's largest association of long-term care and post-acute providers. Over 12,000 profit and non-profit facilities. (4 wds)

15 Travel distance within a smoke barrier must not exceed ____ feet (2 wds)

16 The resources a patient needs and uses. These are based on MDS information. (3 wds)

19 OSHA's summary of occupational injuries/ illnesses must be submitted ______ and posted by the time clock from February to April.

20 In 1946, this Act governs how administrative agencies of the U.S. federal government could propose and establish regulations (2 wds)

22 This program investigates, controls, and prevents infections, chooses procedures to be used, and maintains records of incidences and corrective actions. (2 wds)

24 The inside temperature of a facility must be between ___ and 81 degrees (2 wds)

25 Also called the "purchase journal", this journal includes all purchases made, which will be paid within the next few months (2 wds)

DOWN

2 An Administrator should inform an employee about un upcoming performance evaluation ____ before the evaluation (2 wds)

4 L.L.C. This type of corporation provides liability protection to its owners, but can be taxed as a partnership (3 wds)

6 The instrument that creates a corporation under the laws of the state (3 wds)

7 A written order by a judge, issued on sworn testimony or affidavits supporting probable cause (2 wds)

11 Ownership interest of less than 50% (2 wds)

12 The four financial reports mandated by the GAAP are the balance sheet, the statement of changes in financial position, notes to financial statements and the _____ (2 wds)

14 Center for Health Systems Research and Analysis. Researchers aim to improve long-term care by creating performance measures, and developing information and decision-support systems (5 initials)

17 Using account receivables as security or collateral for a loan

18 Type of ratio that measures debts and assets. The lower the debt ratio, the more financially sound a facility is. (3 wds)

21 During fire drills, the ____ and bedridden are not moved

23 Continuing Care Retirement Community (4 initials)

PUZZLE # 49

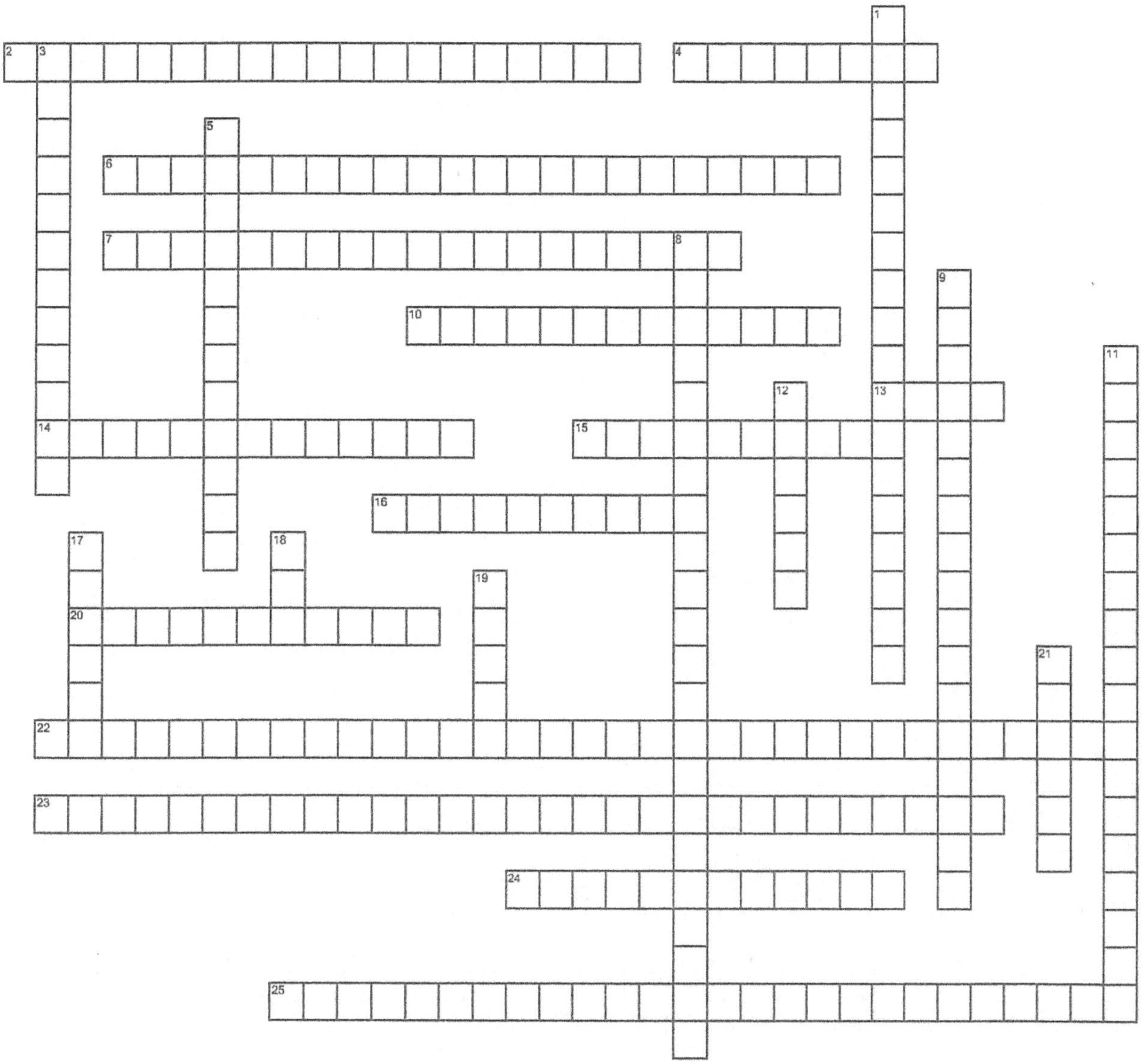

ACROSS

2 A.I.

4 Stored food must be ____ inches from the ceiling

6 T.Q.M. Also called the Continuous Quality Improvement (CQI), a philosophy of total organizational involvement in improving all aspects of quality of service. (3 wds)

7 Who provides the kitchen with a written meal plan for each therapeutic patient diet? (2 wds)

10 This compares investment proposals used in the capital budget. It shows the time it takes for an item to pay for itself. The formula is total investment divided by annual savings (or increased net cash flow) (2 wds)

13 This form of accounting records expenses when cash is dispersed, and revenues when money is received. All are recorded when they occur. Money owed to the facility is not recorded as account receivables, but as revenue after payment is received

14 Rehab, extensive services, special care, clinically complex, and reduced physical function are all examples of _____ (2 wds)

15 This vaccine must be offered, free of charge, to every employee. (2 wds)

16 S.M.A.R.T. stands for specific, ______, attainable, relevant and time-specific

20 A security that represents ownership in a corporation.(2 wds)

22 In 1987, this Act provided criminal penalties for certain acts impacting Medicare and/or Medicaid. Includes the anti-kickback statute. A facility or provider of services cannot induce referrals. (4 wds)

23 S.E.C. A federal agency that regulates financial reporting (4 wds)

24 This ratio measures the long-run liquidity of a facility, or the ability of a facility to meet long-term debts. (this is of interest to would-be creditors) (3 wds)

25 If Medicare owes a facility, they will pay at the end of the year (or require any overpayment to be returned). This is called a _____ Settlement (3 wds)

DOWN

1 The formula average daily census, divided by number of facility beds is called this... (3 wds)

3 The _____ ruled that it is illegal to restrict the advertisement of services or prices, if it results in keeping the public ignorant, or inhibits free flow of information (2 wds)

5 Shares representing ownership of a company. Common and preferred stock a company is authorized to issue, according to their corporate charter. (increasing shares often represents economic health) (2 wds)

8 The principle that all material and relevant facts must be disclosed on financial statements (3 wds)

9 The passage of this Act is considered external feedback of the nursing home industry. It states that inspectors must focus not only on structure (the capacity to give care) and process (the giving of care) but also on outcomes (the results of efforts made) (3 wds)

11 This ratio shows the proportion of revenues earned, to the amount of expenses used to earn those revenues (3 wds)

12 Long-Term Care Facility Improvement Campaign. By the DHHS, in 1976 it supported a comprehensive patient-assessment mechanism, and brought about P.A.C.E. (6 initials)

17 The W-4 form is an required by the IRS. On this form, an employee indicates his or her marital status, and the number of withholding allowances claimed. This information is used by the employer to determine the amount of ____ tax to withhold.

18 Who assigns rates to RUGS? (The rates are adjusted annually for inflation and/or geographic differences) (3 initials)

19 The Health Insurance Portability and Accountability Act, by the Department of Health and Human Services. Enforced privacy rules that a facility must abide to, in order to be eligible for Medicare funds. Provided national standards for Electronic Health Records, as well as national provider ID numbers. (5 initials)

21 The attending physician must have a face-to-face visit with a new resident within ____ days. After that, the physician must see that resident every thirty days for the first three months, and then at sixty-day intervals

PUZZLE # 50

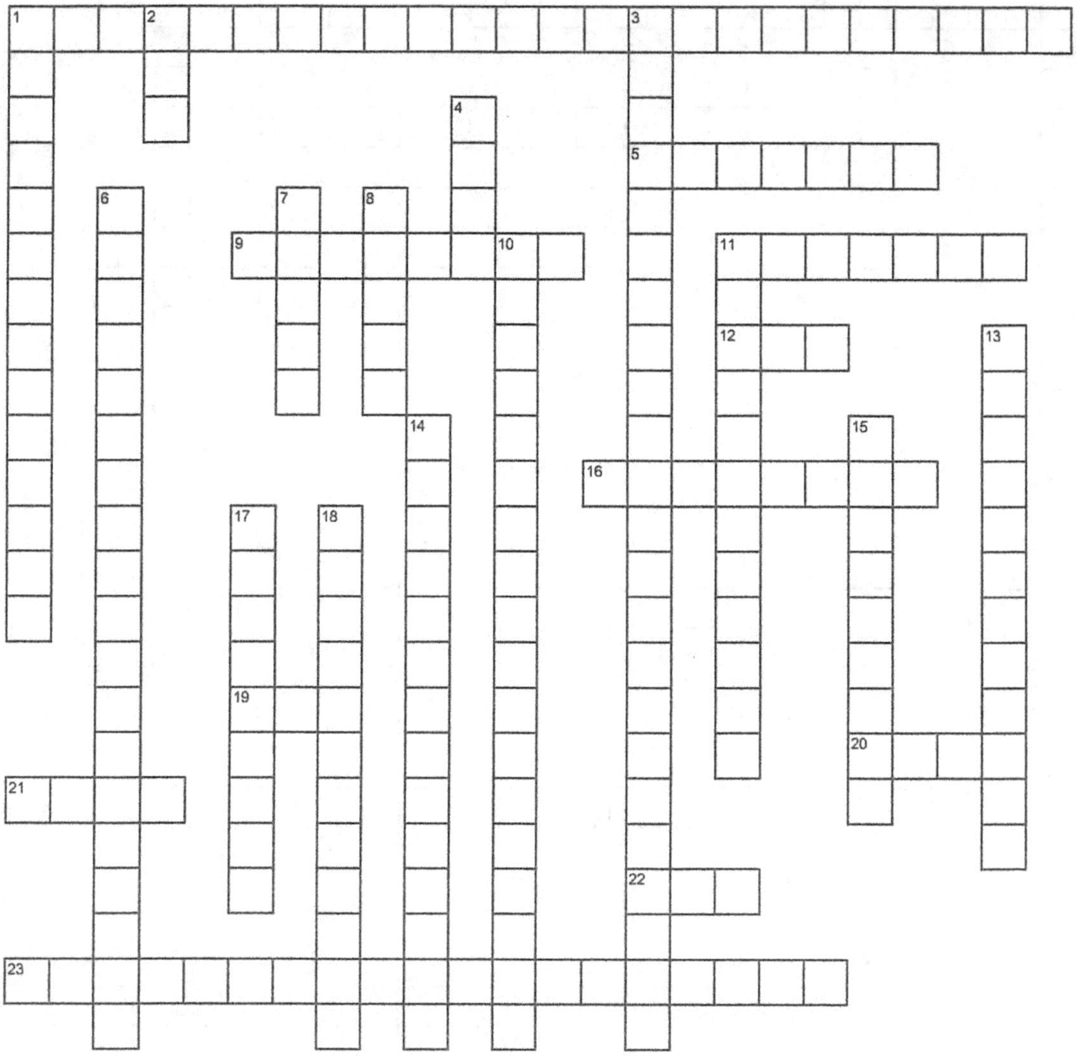

ACROSS

1 P.P.S. Developed for Medicare for skilled nursing facilities. Pays SNF's an all-inclusive rate for all Medicare Part A beneficiary services. Payment is determined by a Case Mix classification system. (3 wds)
5 This form of accounting is GAAP required. Revenues are recorded when earned, expenses are recorded when incurred, regardless of when the transaction occurs. It includes depreciation, account payables and receivables, and prepaid expenses. It provides a clear, accurate picture of a facility's financial position
9 Type of therapy that is geared toward improving ambulation, joint mobility and balance, strength training, fitting and using artificial limbs, and training to use canes or walkers
11 Measures the intensity of care/ services used by a group of residents. Helps classify residents with RUG rates. (2 wds)
12 Stored food must be ___ inches off the floor
16 Home health care is covered by Medicare Part A and Part B, and _____
19 Clear disclaimers in the employee handbook will ____ prevent successful employee lawsuits in court, alleging the handbook to be a binding contract
20 True or false: Food and non-food items must be stored separately
21 Financial Accounts Standards Board. An independent institution that establishes and disseminates the GAAP's principles. (4 initials)
22 Enclosed stairs must have a ___ hour fire resistance.
23 Hepatitis B, Hepatitis C, and HIV/ AIDS are examples of ____ (2 wds)

DOWN

1 A form of managed care, this plan falls between a PPO and HMO. It has some flexibility, charges additional costs for a patient to seek care outside of his or her network, mandates that payment is made when services are rendered, and the consumer must file his or her own claims (3 wds)
2 Satisfaction Assessment Questionaire (3 initials)
3 M.C.O. This type of insurance policy has a limited number of providers, financial incentives for membership, and quality assurance programs. They include HMO's, PPO's, and POS's. (3 wds)
4 Equal Employment Opportunity Commission. For employers of fifteen or more employees, a federal agency that enforces various antidiscrimination laws, and investigates discrimination complaints (4 initials)
6 A summary of an organization's sources and use of cash during an income statement period. A reflection of a firm liquidity. (4 wds)
7 In order to be Medicare eligible for skilled nursing facility care, one must first spend at least ___ days in a hospital, within thirty days of admission into a SNF.
8 A valued resource that benefits a company. It may be current or non-current.
10 Who prescribes a resident's therapeutic diet? (2 wds)
11 C.M.I. Assigns a value to each RUG cell. Part of the RUG factor to calculate a resident's RUG rate (3 wds)
13 Swinging doors must have these (2 wds)
14 M.D.S. Federally legislated, part of the RAI, used in order to do a comprehensive patient assessment. Used for preliminary screenings, to identify potential problems, strengths or preferences. RUG rate is based on this. (3 wds)
15 Money owed/ debt by a company (listed based on due date)
17 Cash activity is grouped into three transaction types: profit-making (operating activities), investing, and ____ (lenders, owners)
18 This type of insurance covers certain forms of care in a skilled nursing facility. It helps cover expenses for days after #100 of Medicare coverage. Covers intermediate care in a facility or at home. Covers care in CCRC's, assisted living facilities and adult day care. Covers custodial care. (3 wds)

PUZZLE # 51

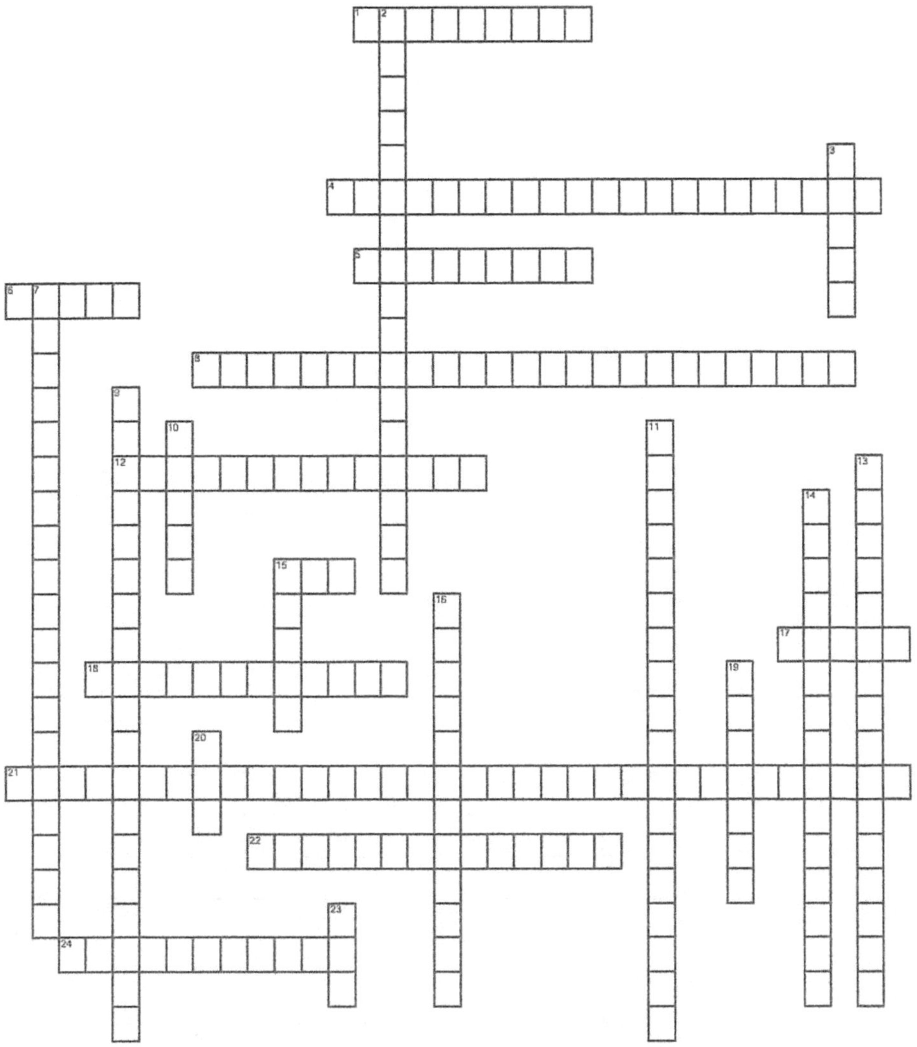

ACROSS

1 Those with Medicare Part A may receive _____ home health visits, at no cost to the patient, if he or she was hospitalized under Medicare Part A, and evaluated to need post-hospital home health care for the final DRG diagnoses

4 A program which induces employers to favor certain disadvantaged people facing barriers to employment, such as welfare recipients or disadvantaged youth. (4 wds)

5 The RUG methodology of assessment classification, where an assessment is placed in the first classification category and where a match is found by evaluating resident conditions and services

6 Enhancements in assets, or reductions in liabilities from outside usual business activities

8 This program, an order from the U.S. President, requires written programs of all contractors with 50 or more employees and $50,000.00 in federal contracts. It is called the Office of ____ (3 wds)

12 Also called preferred shares, a class of ownership, with a higher claim than common stock. A dividend is paid before common stockholders, but shares do not have the same voting rights. (2 wds)

15 According to OSHA, minor injuries or illnesses must be recorded within ___ days

17 By 1935, ___ percent of the aged population were indigent (largely due to the Great Depression)

18 A detailed statement of an organization's financial position. Includes an income statement, balance sheet, statement of cash flows, statement of owner/ shareholder equity, management discussion, an audit opinion, and notes to financial statements. (2 wds)

21 D.H.H.S. A part of the executive branch of government. Concerned with people, and national human concerns. They develop and implement administrative regulations to carry out national health and human services policy objectives. They are the main source of regulations affecting the health care industry. (6 wds)

22 Everyone who receives _____ is approved for Medicare Part A. (2 wds)

24 Which edition of the Life Safety Code of the NFPA must be followed? (2 wds)

DOWN

2 The funds available to a facility.(Current assets less current liabilities) (3 wds)

3 An employee who ignores OSHA rules may be ____

7 A method to measure the potential profitability of an investment (4 wds)

9 When a case regarding an occupational injury or illness is recorded in the log, this form needs to be completed, to include the employee's ID, a description of the event, the injury, and so forth (2 wds)

10 The number of resident groups for RUG's

11 Any injury that is from a work accident or exposure involving a single accident (2 wds)

13 This report, called the Medical Assistance and ____for Medicaid, accompanies payment from public insurers. It lists a resident's name, claim number, service dates, service descriptions, and the total amount billed to the program, specifying allowed and non-allowed charges. (2 wds)

14 Hospice patients may receive Medicare Part A ______ for events unrelated to their terminal illnesses.

15 The Change of Therapy observation period is ___ days, beginning the day following ARD of the resident's last PPS assessment used for payment

16 Another name for an income statement. This statement measures an organization's performance during an accounting period by calculating gross profit, operating income, or net income. (2 wds)

19 The cost of a good or service

20 The 10-K is a required report by ____. It is a more formal and detailed presentation of a company's results, with fewer comments from management. (A 10-Q is similar to a 10-K, but is submitted quarterly) (3 initials)

23 The data needed to assign a patient a RUG rate comes from a subset of items on the ___. It is the standardized, comprehensive assessment form that is completed for every patient in a NF or SNF (3 initials)

PUZZLE # 52

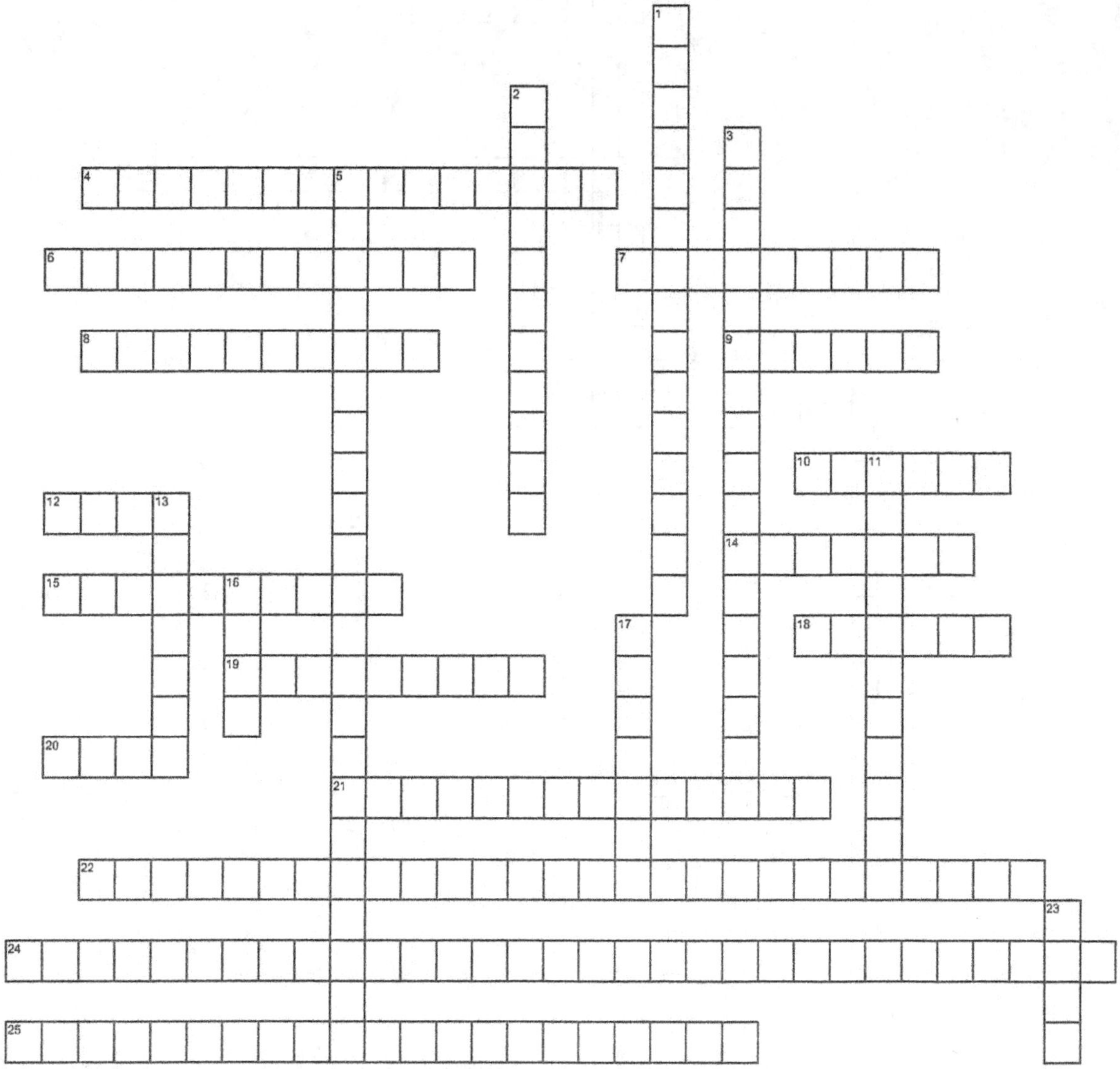

ACROSS

4 The cost of storage, insurance, spoilage and shrinkage or inventory (2 wds)

6 A key factor that can cause movements in bond prices (2 wds)

7 Regarding Medicare patients who have had a hospital stay of three or more days, the day of ____ into a hospital counts toward that three days, but the day of discharge does not.

8 Minimal inventory increases ____ costs. (examples: purchase order preparation, receiving, paying, postage and handling)

9 The four basic elements of an income statement are: revenues, gains, expenses and ____

10 This type of statement provides insight into how well management controls expenses.

12 Program of All-Inclusive Care for Elderly. A DHHS program that supports Medicare and Medicaid enrollees. For members, it becomes the sole source of services, but members may leave the program at any time. This was brought about by the Long-Term Care Facility Improvement Campaign. (4 initials)

14 Earnings from usual business activities

15 The daily rate that a facility is paid for a Medicare Part A resident depends on which of ___ RUG's that patient is assigned (2 wds)

18 Provided a Medicare patient is approved, their first ___ days in a nursing facility are covered by insurance

19 The Management's Discussion and Analysis of operations (MD&A) is the _____ portion of the annual report. It provides an overview of the previous years operation and financial performance, and outlines future goals and directions.

20 Federal Unemployment Tax Act

21 Type of statement that shows funds available to a facility, and is used to measure a company's efficiency and short-term financial health. (2 wds)

22 In 1970, this Act focused on safety standards. Enforced by each state, states were permitted to establish their own inspection programs and industrial safety labs

24 H.C.F.A. They administer Medicare and Medicaid, and write the federal requirements for nursing facilities and skilled nursing facilities.(4 wds)

25 After a patient assessment is completed, a _____ must be done within seven days (3 wds)

DOWN

1 The distance between a door in any room, and exit access must not exceed ____ feet

2 This term describes revenue minus the cost of goods sold (in other words, revenue after production costs). Can be used toward operating expenses (2 wds)

3 S.S.A. A response to the growing number of poor people. An "old-age" assurance policy. This Act is responsible for generating financial support for older people, and causing growth in nursing facility care. (3 wds)

5 These are given in rural settings, or when the mandatory amount of nurses are not needed in a NF. If one is approved, there must be a nurse or doctor who can respond to calls 24/7. They are approved by CMS, and subject to annual review. (3 wds)

11 A Registered Nurse must be present at a NF/ SNF for eight _____ hours a day, seven days a week

13 End of Therapy- Other Medicare Required Assessment (7 initials) Must be completed when a patient does not receive therapy services for three consecutive days.

16 True or false: Capital expenditures must be tangible assets, have a minimal useful life of over one year, and meet minimum monetary cutoff in accordance with an organization's policy.

17 Any new rooms added to U.S. hospitals must be _____ rooms

23 A fixed income security. It is used to raise capital for building or renovations. It is a loan from a lender, from a bank or investor, where the lender gets interest payments until the maturity date.

PUZZLE # 53

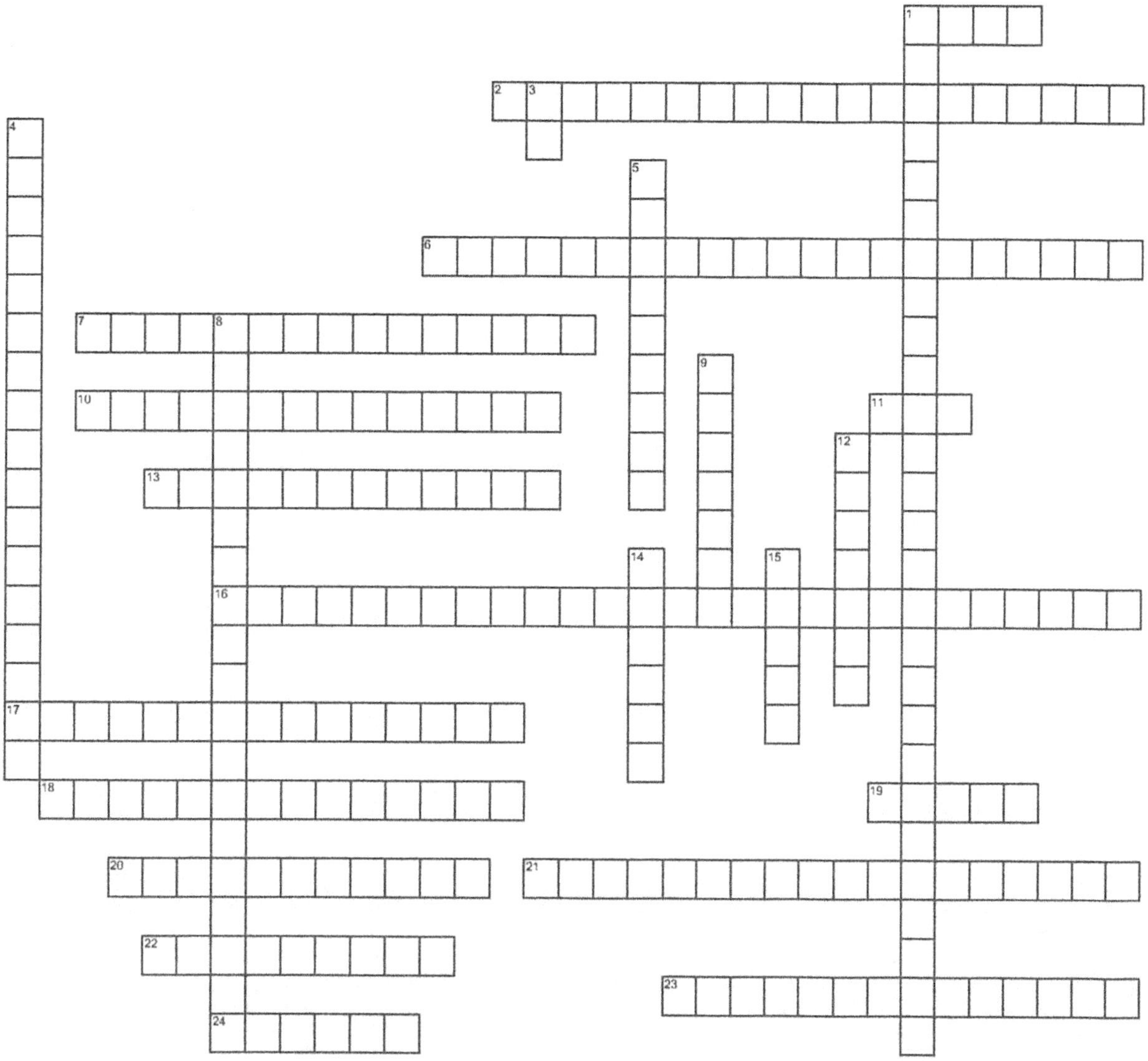

ACROSS

1 A set of items or responses from an MDS that are indicators of a particular issue or condition that effects a resident. These bring attention to what merits additional review or assessment. (4 initials)

2 P.H.S. It coordinates with states to set and implement a national health policy, and pursues effective inter-governmental relations. Used for research, prevention and control of diseases, the development of health resources, alcohol and substance abuse, drug safety, safe food handling, and medical device safety. (3 wds)

6 A.O.A. A part of the Human Development Services department of DHHS. It is a major resource for legislation, policy and funding. Promotes welfare for those age 60+. (3 wds)

7 This form must be signed 48 hours before a Medicare resident is discharged. The original goes to the Medical Billing department, and a copy is added to the patient's chart. The resident or family member may appeal this form, but they must acknowledge the last covered day. (There is no charge the date of discharge, because no skilled services are provided that day) (2 wds)

10 Upholstered furniture and mattresses must be ___ (2 wds)

11 Nursing time schedule records are maintained for ___ year(s)

13 Always ensure the integration of ____perspectives in order to maximize resident quality of life, and quality of care.

16 An organized panel set up to administer the process under the National Labor Relations Act, under which unions become certified as the bargaining agents for groups of workers (4 wds)

17 This Law penalizes anyone who knowingly solicits, receives offers or pays remuneration in cash or in king, for referrals. (3 wds)

18 Evidence has shown that care is most successful if it is _________

19 A full-time Registered Nurse may be the charge nurse if there are less than ___ beds in a facility

20 This Act prohibits discrimination in hiring, firing, promotion, transfer, and admission to training programs. It applies to employers with fifteen or more employees. It is implemented by the EEOC (Equal Employment Opportunities Commission). (2 wds)

21 Cash from ____ involves the purchase and sale of long-term assets such as property, plant and equipment, as well as the investment of one company into another (2 wds)

22 Linen or trash containers must be limited to a ___ gallon capacity in any 64 square foot area. (2 wds)

23 L.C.D.

24 A facility purchases a ____ bond if handling and managing patient funds

DOWN

1 Transactions that generate new funds from investors, banks and shareholders, or returned funds to these parties. (Significant to investors, since it allows them to evaluate how viable a company is, short-term, and provides an assessment of its ability to pay its bills (4 wds)

3 Unemployment Compensation. The Social Security Act of 1935 started this program. It provides temporary and partial wage replacement to the involuntarily unemployed, and helps stabilize the economy during recessions. (2 initials)

4 Funds for unemployment compensation come from a ____ based on wages of each employee, up to a certain maximum. (3 wds)

5 Type of summary that includes a list of services delivered to a resident, goals achieved, and post-discharge planning. It becomes a part of the medical record.

8 Inflows and outflows of cash that result from an organization's sale of services is called cash from ___ (2 wds)

9 Claiming this type of work environment requires evidence of pervasive, offensive conduct of a sexual nature.

12 When a dual-eligible resident (Medicare and Medicaid) receives this level of care (for terminally ill) at a skilled nursing facility, ____ is responsible for all care, and receives a per diem payment from Medicare.

14 Cash flow from ___ equals operating activities

15 This Medicare insurance covers inpatient hospital services, skilled nursing care, home health care and hospice. For residents with this type of Medicare, bills are submitted for each patient, and sent to a fiscal intermediary (one bill per patient) (2 wds)

PUZZLE

SOLUTIONS

PUZZLE # 1

Solution:

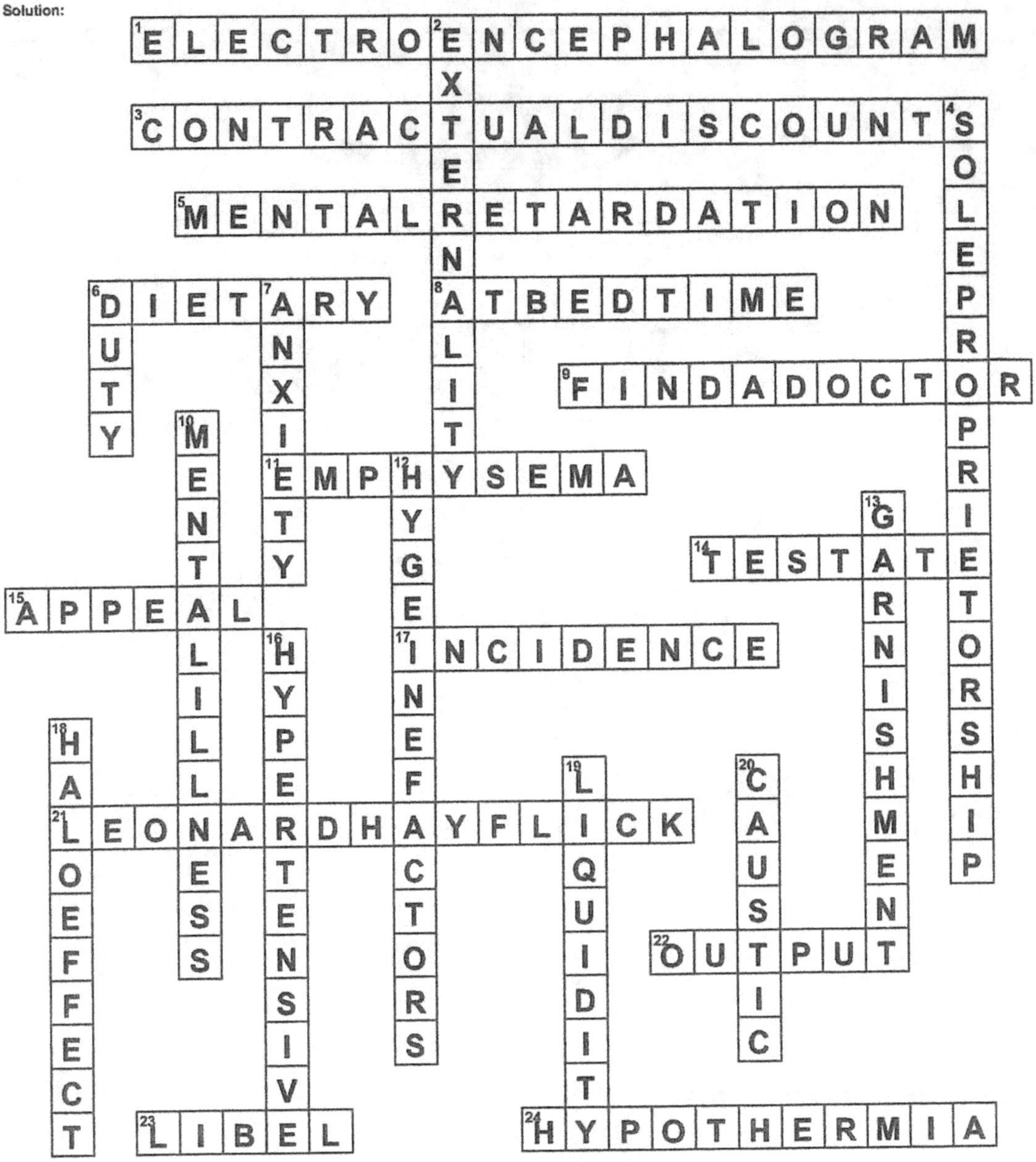
1 ELECTROENCEPHALOGRAM
2 EXTERNALITIT
3 CONTRACTUALDISCOUNTS
4 SOLEPROPRIETORSHIP
5 MENTALRETARDATION
6 DIETARY
6 DUTY
7 ANXIETY
8 ATBEDTIME
9 FINDADOCTOR
10 MENTALILLNESS
11 EMPHYSEMA
12 HYGIENEFACTORS
13 GARNISHMENT
14 TESTATE
15 APPEAL
16 HYPERTENSIVE
17 INCIDENCE
18 HALOEFFECT
19 LIQUIDITY
20 CAUSTIC
21 LEONARDHAYFLICK
22 OUTPUT
23 LIBEL
24 HYPOTHERMIA

PUZZLE # 2

Solution:

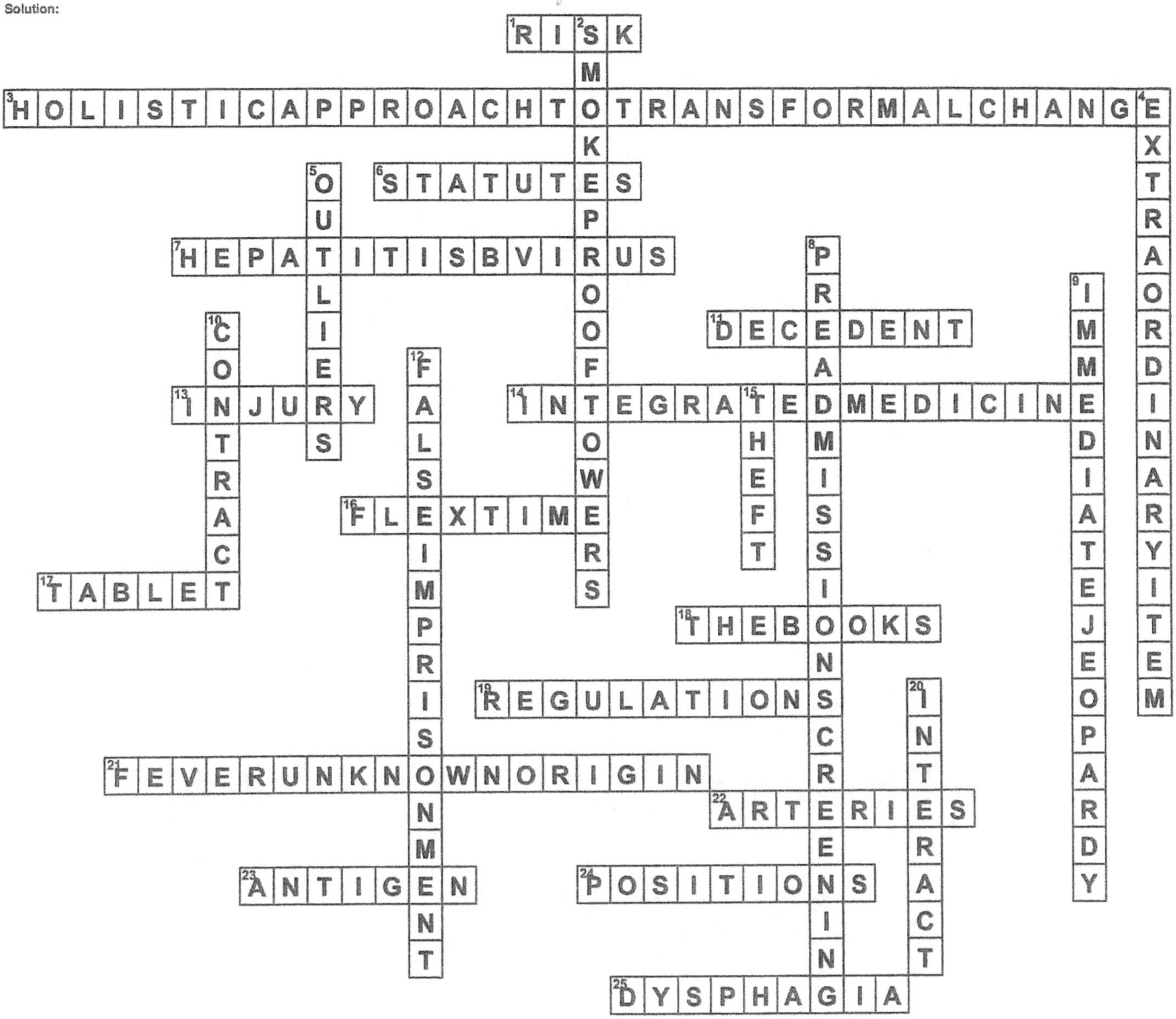
1 RISK
2 SMOKEPROOFTOWERS
3 HOLISTICAPPROACHTOTRANSFORMALCHANGE
4 EXTRAORDINARYITEM
5 OUTLIERS
6 STATUTES
7 HEPATITISBVIRUS
8 PREADMISSIONSCREENING
9 IMMEDIATEJEOPARDY
10 CONTRACT
11 DECEDENT
12 FALSEIMPRISONMENT
13 INJURY
14 INTEGRATEDMEDICINE
15 THEFT
16 FLEXTIME
17 TABLET
18 THEBOOKS
19 REGULATIONS
20 INTERACT
21 FEVERUNKNOWNORIGIN
22 ARTERIES
23 ANTIGEN
24 POSITIONS
25 DYSPHAGIA

PUZZLE # 3

Solution:

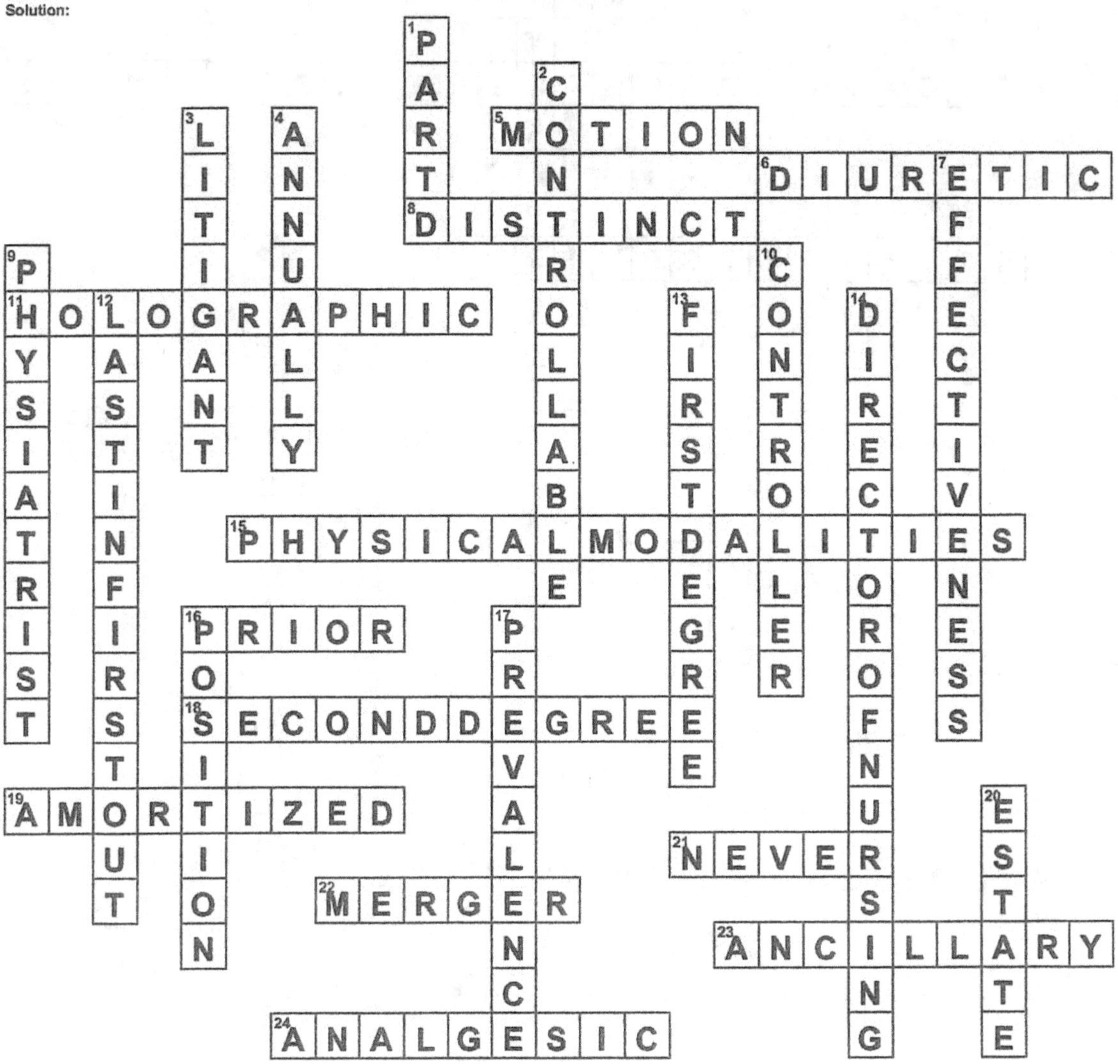

1 PART
2 CONTROLLABLE
3 LITIGANT
4 ANNUALLY
5 MOTION
6 DIURETIC
7 EFFECTIVENESS
8 DISTINCT
9 PHYSIATRIST
10 CONTROLLER
11 HOLOGRAPHIC
12 LASTINFIRSTOUT
13 FIRSTDEGREE
14 DIRECTOROFNURSING
15 PHYSICALMODALITIES
16 PRIOR
16 POSITION
17 PREVALENCE
18 SECONDDEGREE
19 AMORTIZED
20 ESTATE
21 NEVER
22 MERGER
23 ANCILLARY
24 ANALGESIC

PUZZLE # 4

Solution:

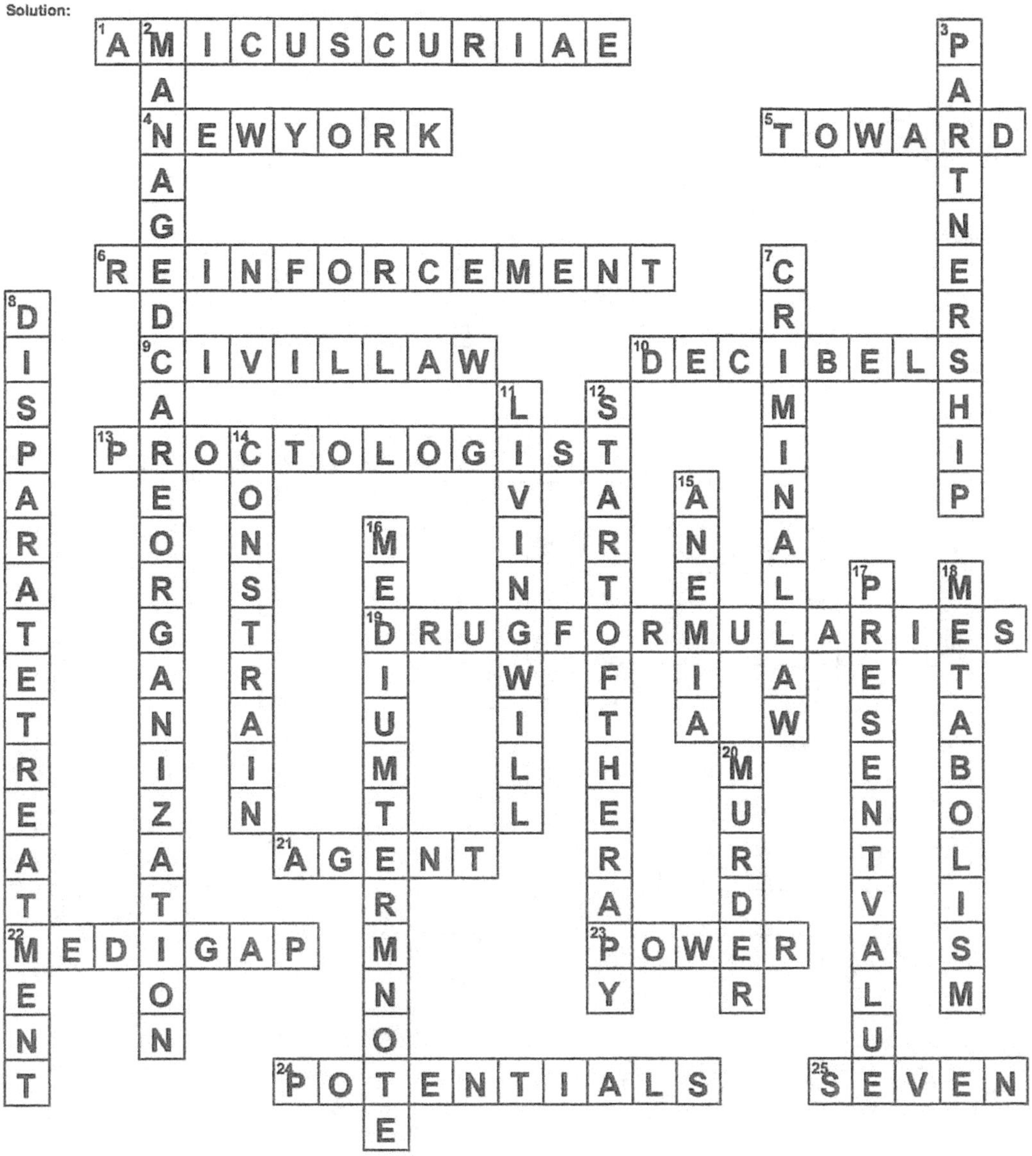
1 AMICUSCURIAE
2 MANAGEDCAREORGANIZATION
3 PARTNERSHIP
4 NEWYORK
5 TOWARD
6 REINFORCEMENT
7 CRIMINALLAW
8 DISPARATETREATMENT
9 CIVILLAW
10 DECIBELS
11 LIVINGWILL
12 STARTOFTHERAPY
13 PROCTOLOGIST
14 CONSTRAIN
15 ANEMIA
16 MEDIUMTERMNOTE
17 PRESENTVALUE
18 METABOLISM
19 DRUGFORMULARIES
20 MURDER
21 AGENT
22 MEDIGAP
23 POWER
24 POTENTIALS
25 SEVEN

PUZZLE # 5

Solution:

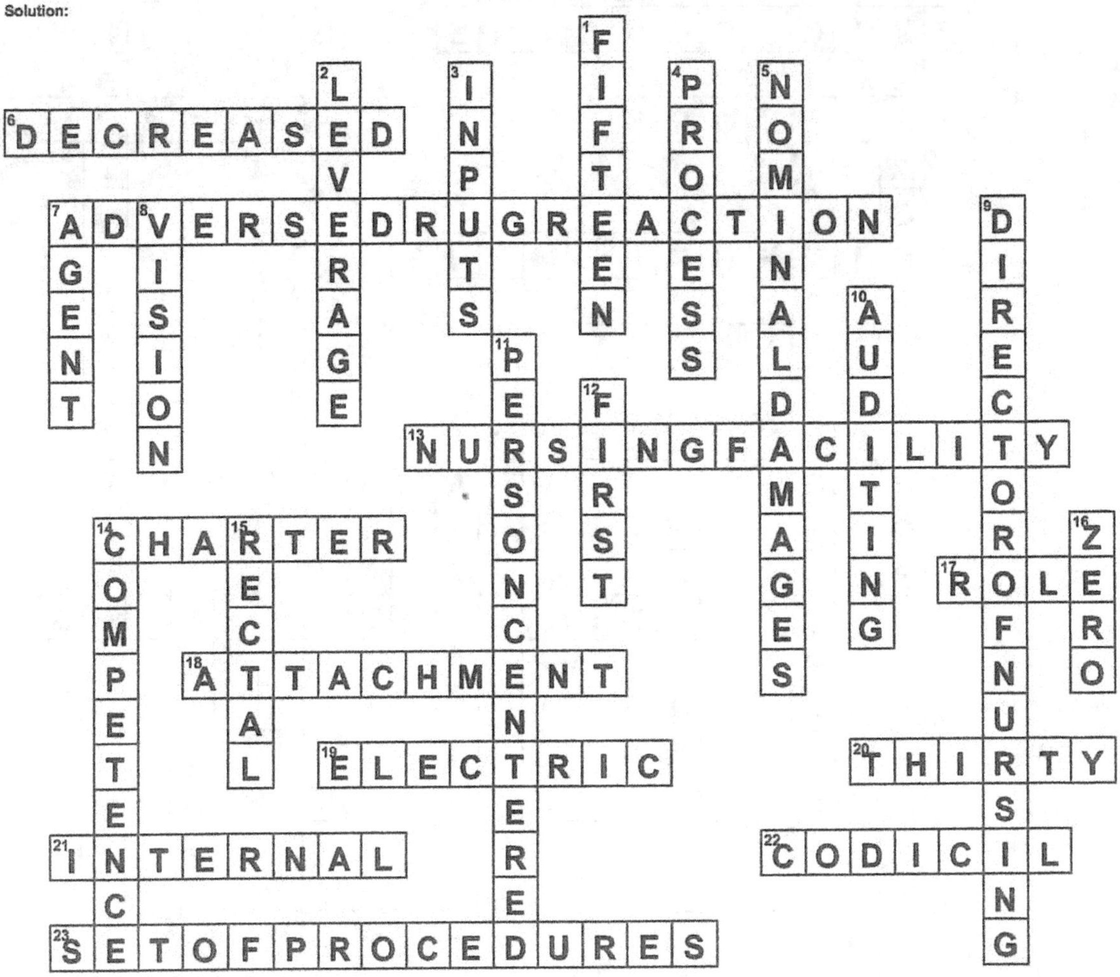
1 FIFTEEN
2 LEVERAGE
3 INPUTS
4 PROCESS
5 NOMINALDAMAGES
6 DECREASED
7 ADVERSEDRUGREACTION
7 AGENT
8 VISION
9 DIRECTOROFNURSING
10 AUDITING
11 PERSONCENTERED
12 FIRST
13 NURSINGFACILITY
14 CHARTER
14 COMPETENCE
15 RECTAL
16 ZERO
17 ROLE
18 ATTACHMENT
19 ELECTRIC
20 THIRTY
21 INTERNAL
22 CODICIL
23 SETOFPROCEDURES

PUZZLE # 6

Solution:

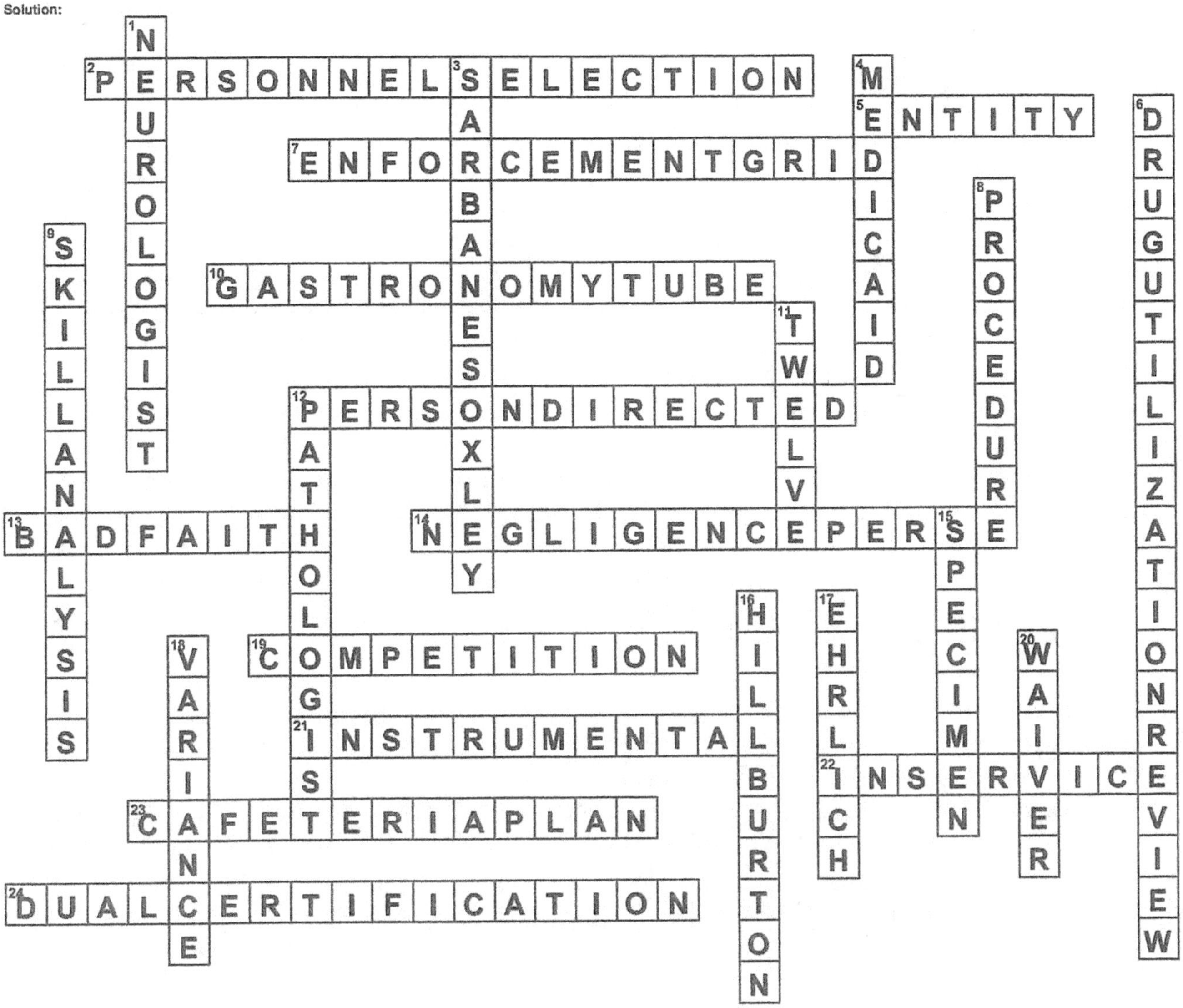
1 NEUROLOGIST
2 PERSONNELSELECTION
3 SARBANESOXLEY
4 MEDICAID
5 ENTITY
6 DRUGUTILIZATIONREVIEW
7 ENFORCEMENTGRID
8 PROCEDURE
9 SKILLANALYSIS
10 GASTRONOMYTUBE
11 TWELVE
12 PERSONDIRECTED
12 PATHOLOGIS
13 BADFAITH
14 NEGLIGENCEPERSE
15 SPECIMEN
16 HILLBURTON
17 EHRLICH
18 VARIANCE
19 COMPETITION
20 WAIVER
21 INSTRUMENTAL
22 INSERVICE
23 CAFETERIAPLAN
24 DUALCERTIFICATION

PUZZLE # 7

Solution:

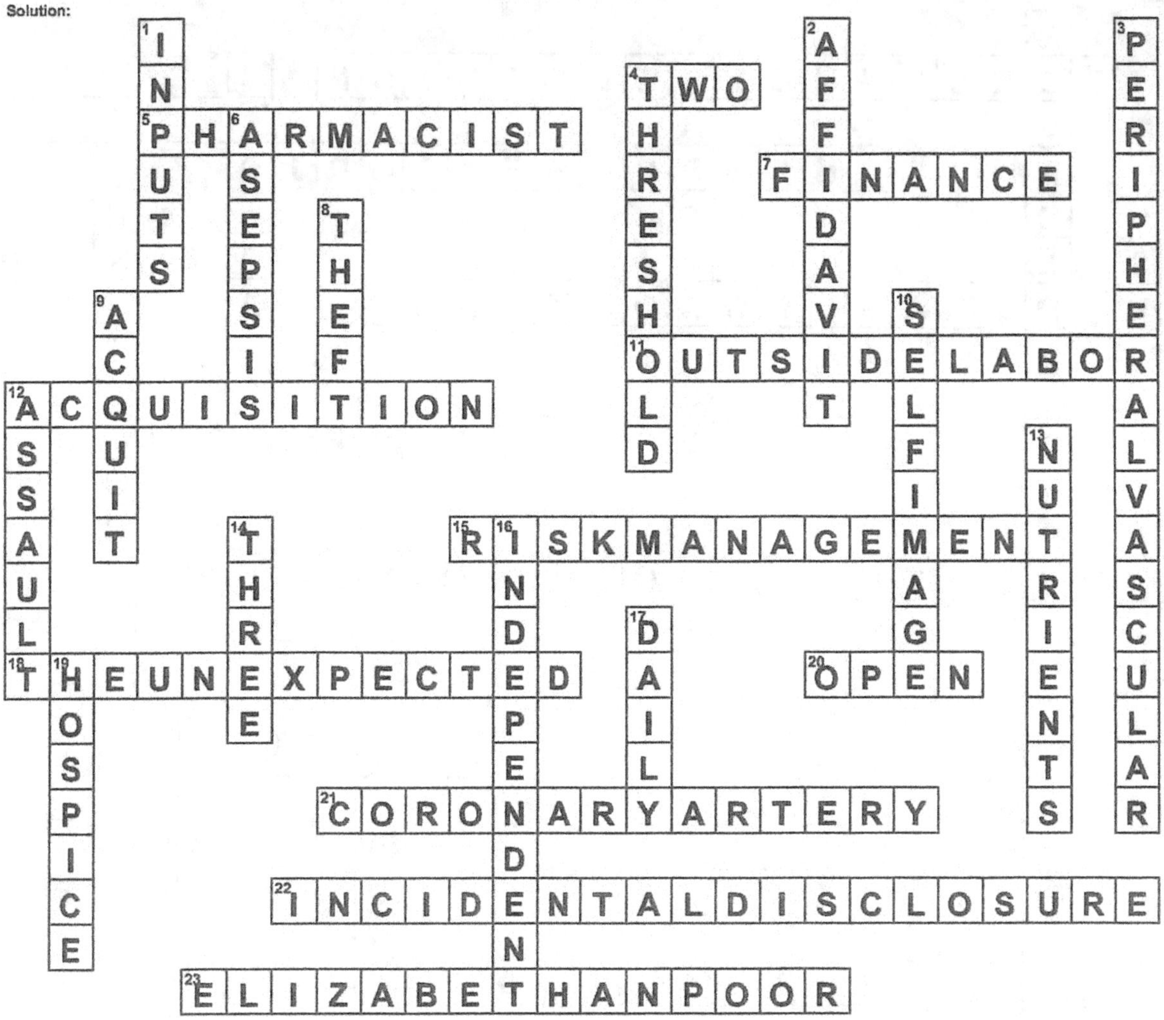

1 INPUTS
2 AFFIDAVIT
3 PERIPHERALVASCULAR
4 TWO
4 THRESHOLD
5 PHARMACIST
6 ASEPSIS
7 FINANCE
8 THEFT
9 ACQUIT
10 SELFIMAGE
11 OUTSIDELABOR
12 ACQUISITION
12 ASSAULT
13 NUTRIENTS
14 THREE
15 RISKMANAGEMENT
16 INDEPENDENT
17 DAIL
18 THEUNEXPECTED
19 HOSPICE
20 OPEN
21 CORONARYARTERY
22 INCIDENTALDISCLOSURE
23 ELIZABETHANPOOR

PUZZLE # 8

Solution:

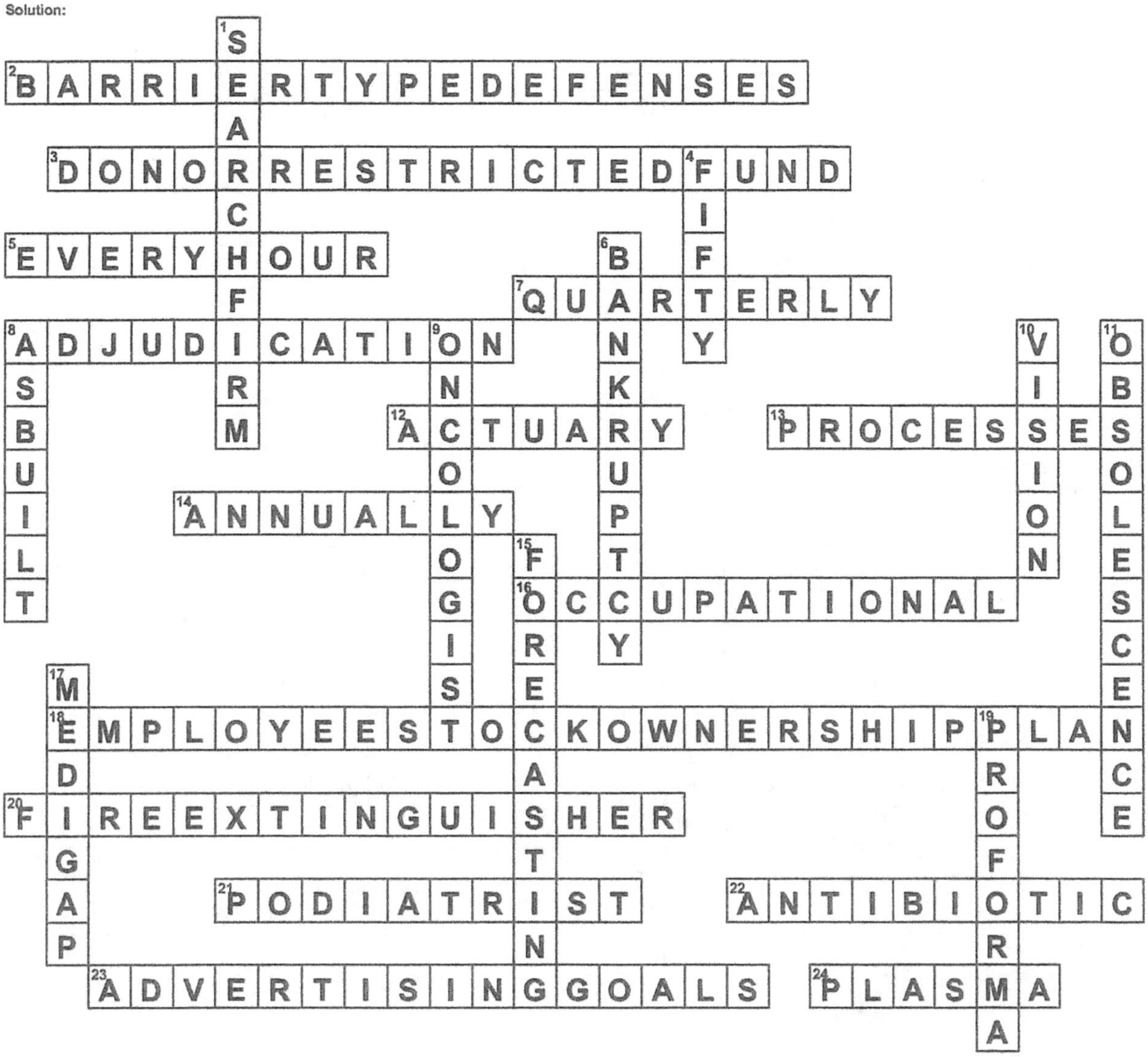

1 SEARCHFIRM
2 BARRIERTYPEDEFENSES
3 DONORRESTRICTEDFUND
4 FIFTY
5 EVERYHOUR
6 BANKRUPTCY
7 QUARTERLY
8 ADJUDICATION
8 ASBUILT
9 ONCOLOGIST
10 VISION
11 OBSOLESCENCE
12 ACTUARY
13 PROCESSES
14 ANNUALLY
15 FORECASTING
16 OCCUPATIONAL
17 MEDIGAP
18 EMPLOYEESTOCKOWNERSHIPPLAN
19 PROFORMA
20 FIREEXTINGUISHER
21 PODIATRIST
22 ANTIBIOTIC
23 ADVERTISINGGOALS
24 PLASMA

PUZZLE # 9

Solution:

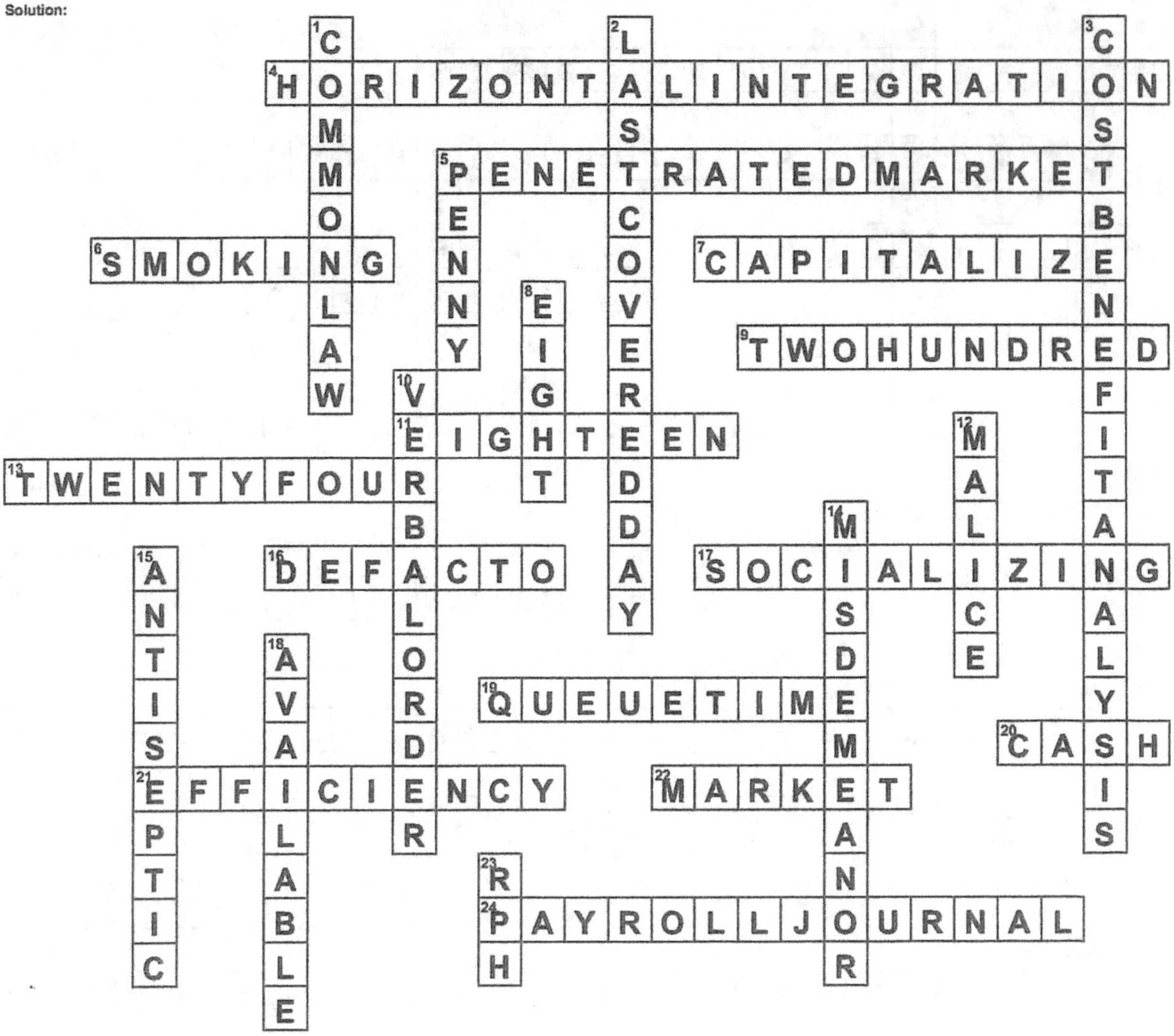

1 COMMONLAW
2 LASTCOVEREDDAY
3 COSTBENEFITANALYSIS
4 HORIZONTALINTEGRATION
5 PENETRATEDMARKET
PENNY
6 SMOKING
7 CAPITALIZE
8 EIGHT
9 TWOHUNDRED
10 VERBALORDER
11 EIGHTEEN
12 MALICE
13 TWENTYFOUR
14 MISDEMEANOR
15 ANTISEPTIC
16 DEFACTO
17 SOCIALIZING
18 AVAILABLE
19 QUEUETIME
20 CASH
21 EFFICIENCY
22 MARKET
23 RPH
24 PAYROLLJOURNAL

PUZZLE # 10

Solution:

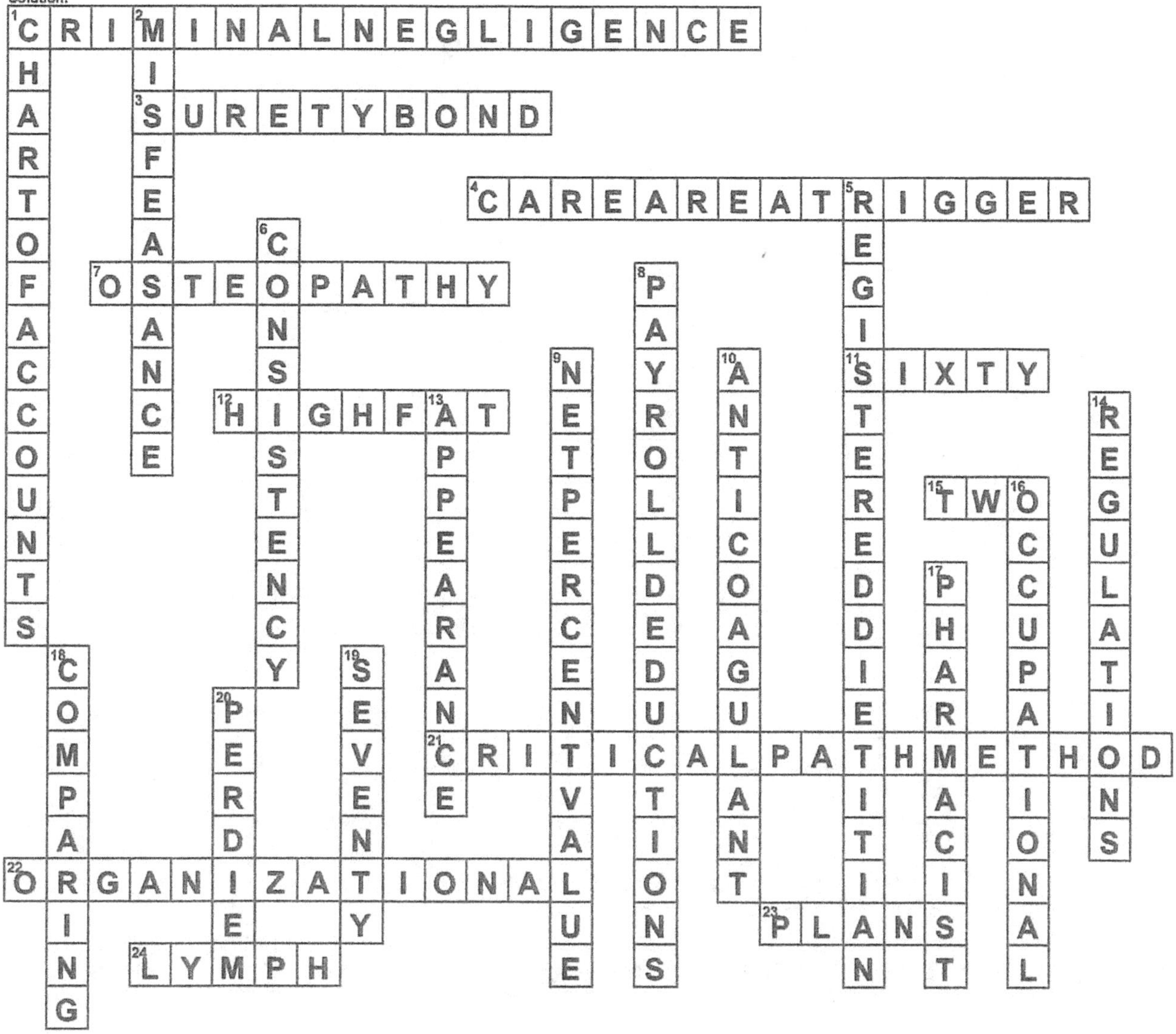

1 CRIMINALNEGLIGENCE
2 MISFEASANCE
3 SURETYBOND
4 CAREAREATRIGGER
5 REGISTEREDDIETITIAN
6 CONSISTENCY
7 OSTEOPATHY
8 PAYROLLDEDUCTIONS
9 NETPERCENTVALUE
10 ANTICOAGULANT
11 SIXTY
12 HIGHFAT
13 APPEARANCE
14 REGULATIONS
15 TWO
16 OCCUPATIONAL
17 PHARMACIST
18 COMPARING
19 SEVENTY
20 PERDIEM
21 CRITICALPATHMETHOD
22 ORGANIZATIONAL
23 PLANS
24 LYMPH
1 CHARTOFACCOUNTS

PUZZLE # 11

Solution:

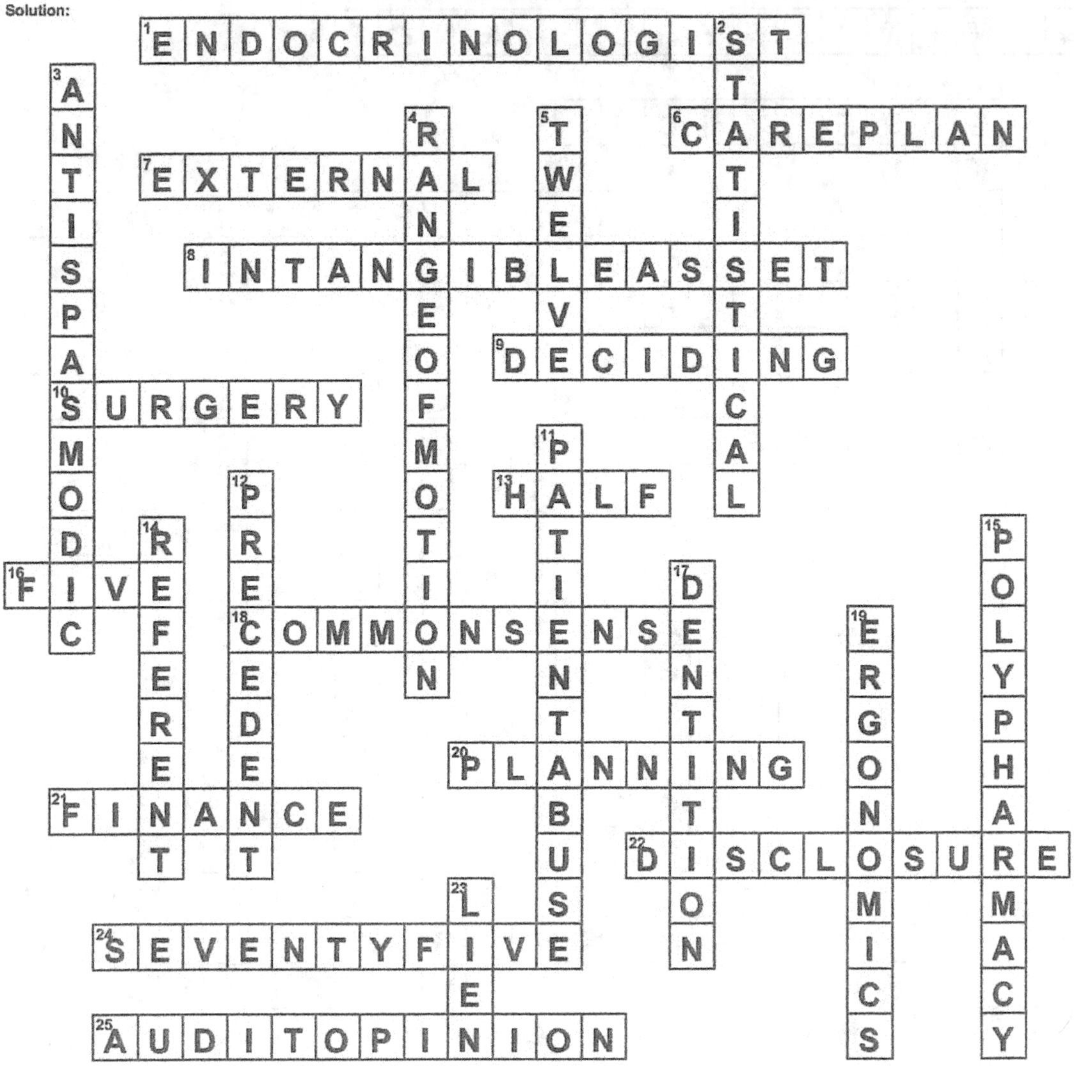
1 ENDOCRINOLOGIST
2 STATISTICAL
3 ANTISPASMODIC
4 RANGEOFMOTION
5 TWELVE
6 CAREPLAN
7 EXTERNAL
8 INTANGIBLEASSET
9 DECIDING
10 SURGERY
11 PATIENTABUSE
12 PRECEDENT
13 HALF
14 REFERENT
15 POLYPHARMACY
16 FIVE
17 DENTITION
18 COMMONSENSE
19 ERGONOMICS
20 PLANNING
21 FINANCE
22 DISCLOSURE
23 LIES
24 SEVENTYFIVE
25 AUDITOPINION

PUZZLE # 12

Solution:

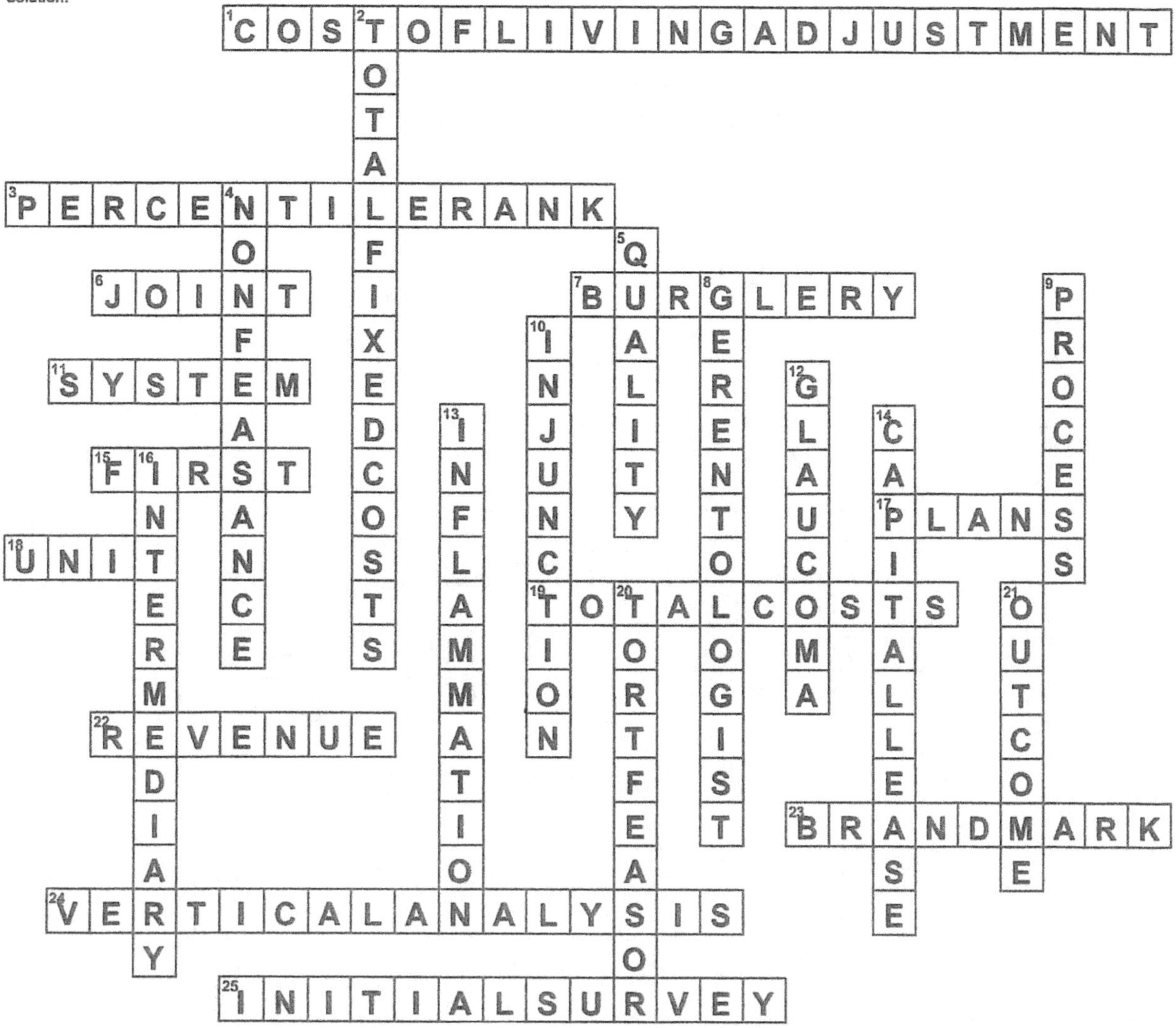

1 COSTOFLIVINGADJUSTMENT
2 TOTALFIXEDCOSTS
3 PERCENTILERANK
4 NONFEASANCE
5 QUALITY
6 JOINT
7 BURGLERY
8 GERENTOLOGIST
9 PROCESS
10 INJUNCTION
11 SYSTEM
12 GLAUCOMA
13 INFLAMMATION
14 CAPITALLEASE
15 FIRST
16 INTERMEDIARY
17 PLANS
18 UNIT
19 TOTALCOSTS
20 TORTFEASOR
21 OUTCOME
22 REVENUE
23 BRANDMARK
24 VERTICALANALYSIS
25 INITIALSURVEY

PUZZLE # 13

Solution:

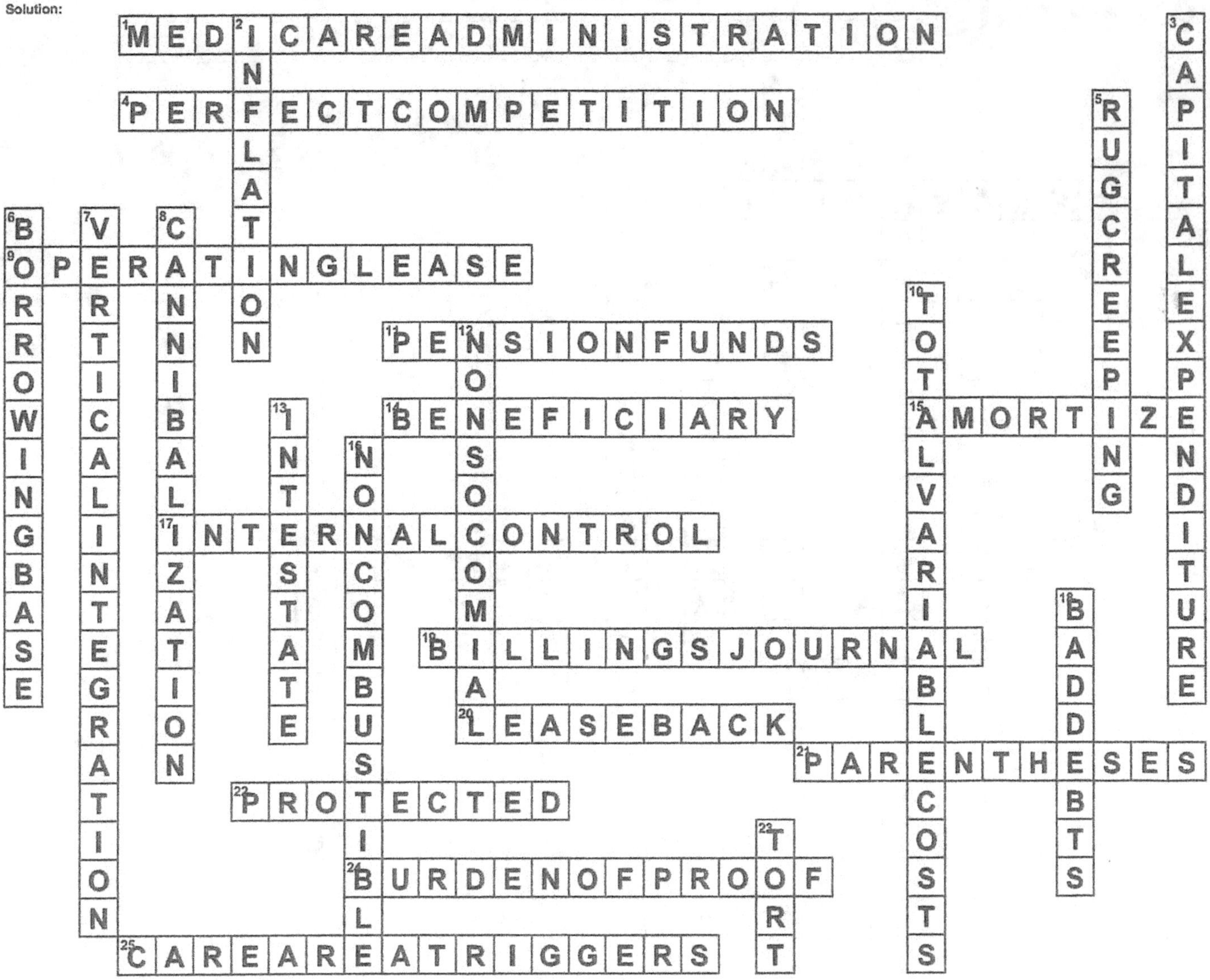
1 MEDICAREADMINISTRATION
2 INFLATION
3 CAPITALEXPENDITURE
4 PERFECTCOMPETITION
5 RUGCREEPING
6 BORROWINGBASE
7 VERTICALINTEGRATION
8 CANNIBALIZATION
9 OPERATINGLEASE
10 TOTALVARIABLECOSTS
11 PENSIONFUNDS
12 NONSOCOMIAL
13 INTERSTATE
14 BENEFICIARY
15 AMORTIZE
16 NONCOMBUSTIBLE
17 INTERNALCONTROL
18 BADDEBTS
19 BILLINGSJOURNAL
20 LEASEBACK
21 PARENTHESES
22 PROTECTED
23 TORT
24 BURDENOFPROOF
25 CAREAREATRIGGERS

PUZZLE # 14

Solution:

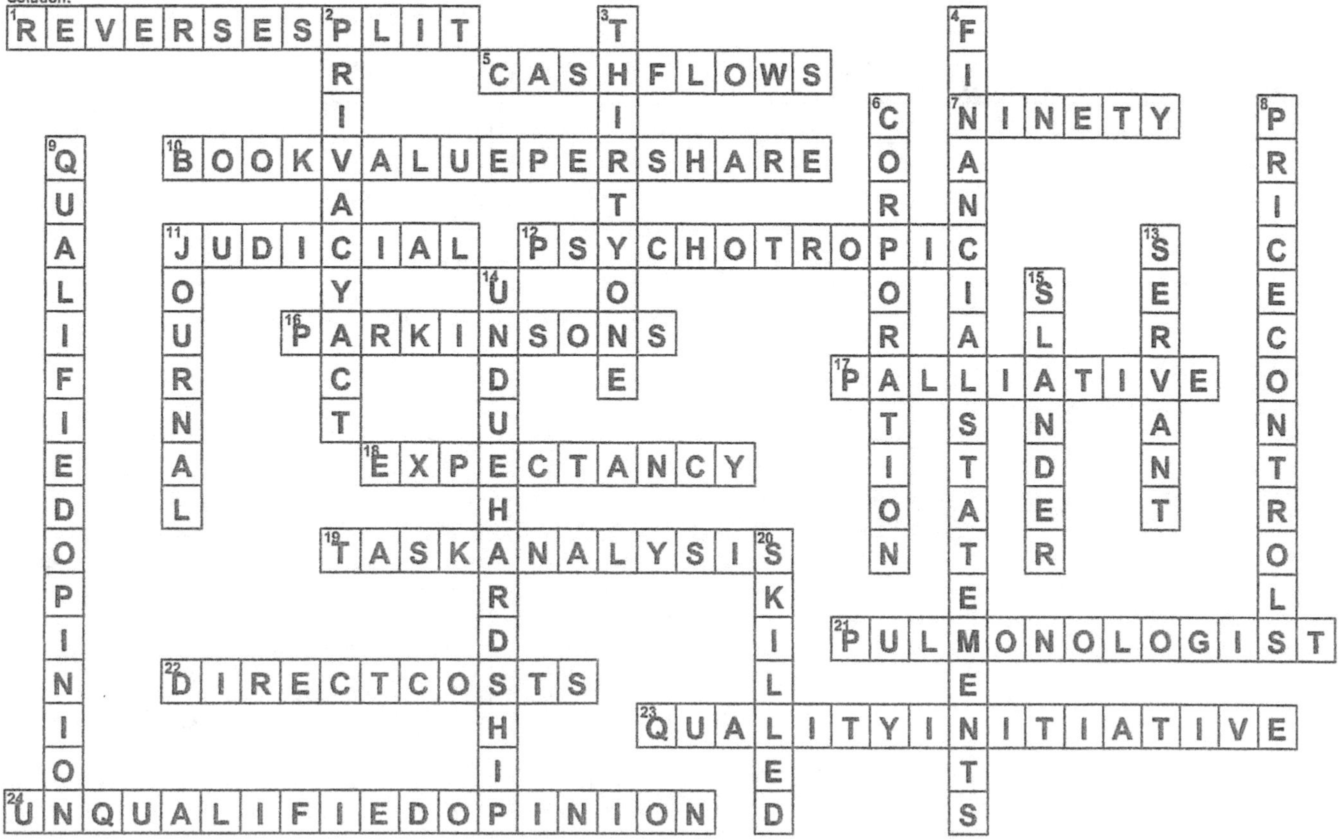
1 REVERSESPLIT
2 PRIVACYACT
3 THIRTYONE
4 FINANCIALSTATEMENTS
5 CASHFLOWS
6 CORPORATION
7 NINETY
8 PRICECONTROL
9 QUALIFIEDOPINION
10 BOOKVALUEPERSHARE
11 JUDICIAL
11 JOURNAL
12 PSYCHOTROPIC
13 SERVANT
14 UNDUEHARDSHIP
15 SLANDER
16 PARKINSONS
17 PALLIATIVE
18 EXPECTANCY
19 TASKANALYSIS
20 SKILLED
21 PULMONOLOGIST
22 DIRECTCOSTS
23 QUALITYINITIATIVE
24 UNQUALIFIEDOPINION

PUZZLE # 15

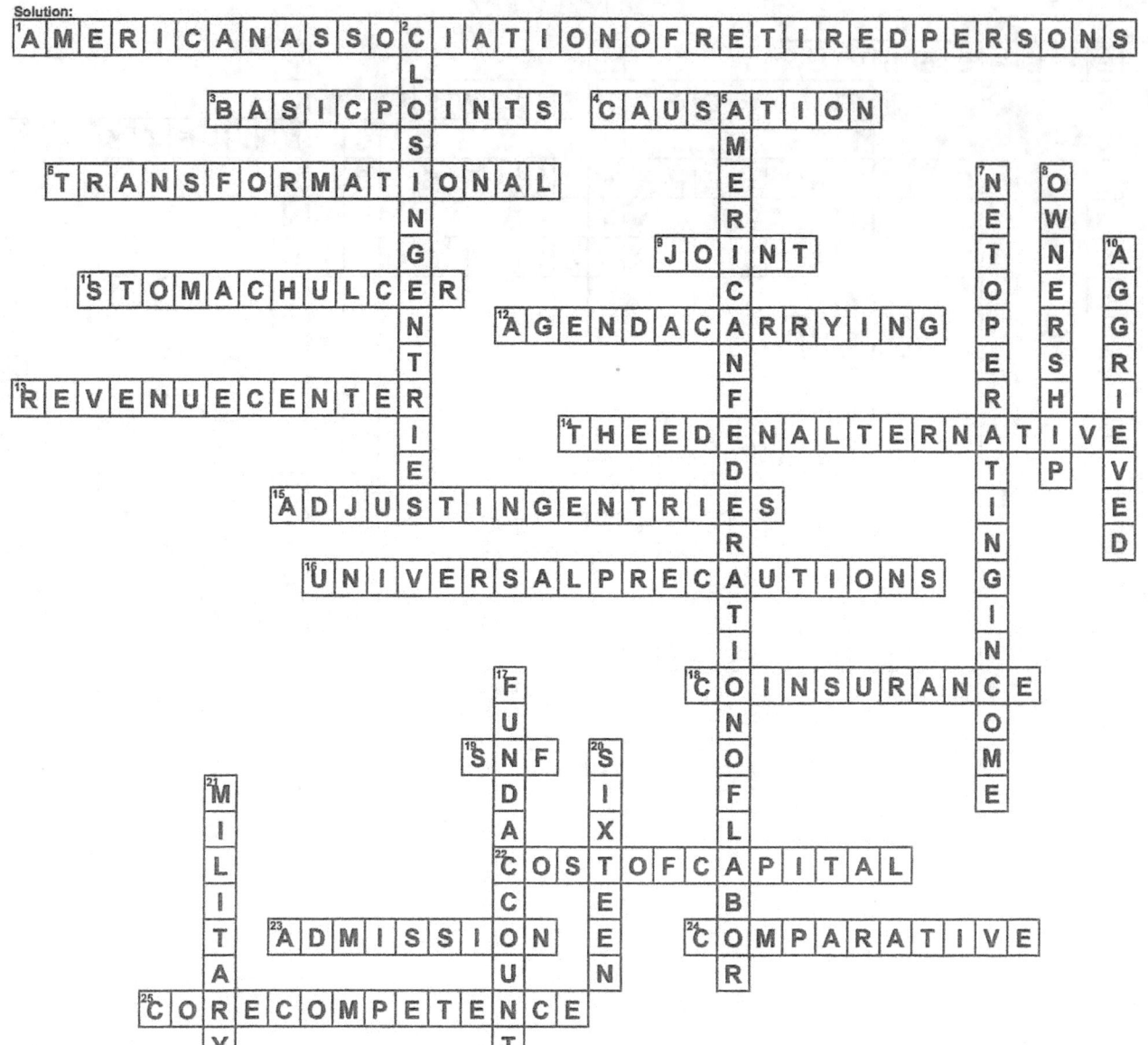

Solution:

Across

1. AMERICANASSOCIATIONOFRETIREDPERSONS
3. BASICPOINTS
4. CAUSATION
6. TRANSFORMATIONAL
9. JOINT
11. STOMACHULCER
12. AGENDACARRYING
13. REVENUECENTER
14. THEEDENALTERNATIVE
15. ADJUSTINGENTRIES
16. UNIVERSALPRECAUTIONS
18. COINSURANCE
19. SNF
22. COSTOFCAPITAL
23. ADMISSION
24. COMPARATIVE
25. CORECOMPETENCE

Down

2. CLOSINGENTRIES
5. AMERICANFEDERATIONOFLABOR
7. NETOPERATINGINCOME
8. OWNERSHIP
10. AGGRIEVED
17. FUNDACCOUNT
20. SIXTEEN
21. MILITARY

PUZZLE # 16

Solution:

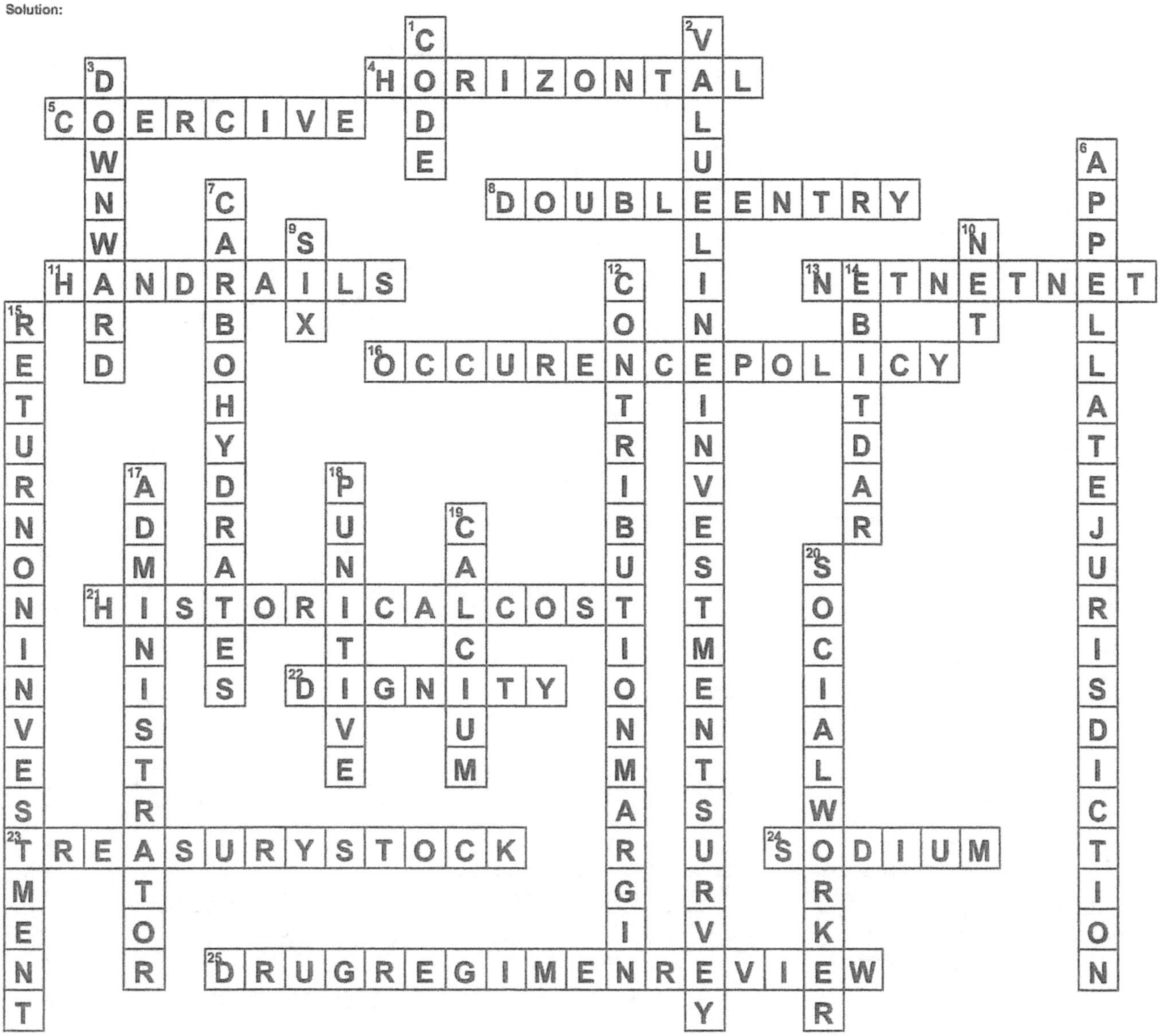

1 CODE
2 VALUELINEINVESTMENTSURVEY
3 DOWNWARD
4 HORIZONTAL
5 COERCIVE
6 APPELLATEJURISDICTION
7 CARBOHYDRATES
8 DOUBLEENTRY
9 SIX
10 NET
11 HANDRAILS
12 CONTRIBUTIONMARGIN
13 NETNETNET
14 EBITDAR
15 RETURNONINVESTMENT
16 OCCURENCEPOLICY
17 ADMINISTRATOR
18 PUNITIVE
19 CALCIUM
20 SOCIALWORKER
21 HISTORICALCOST
22 DIGNITY
23 TREASURYSTOCK
24 SODIUM
25 DRUGREGIMENREVIEW

PUZZLE # 17

Solution:

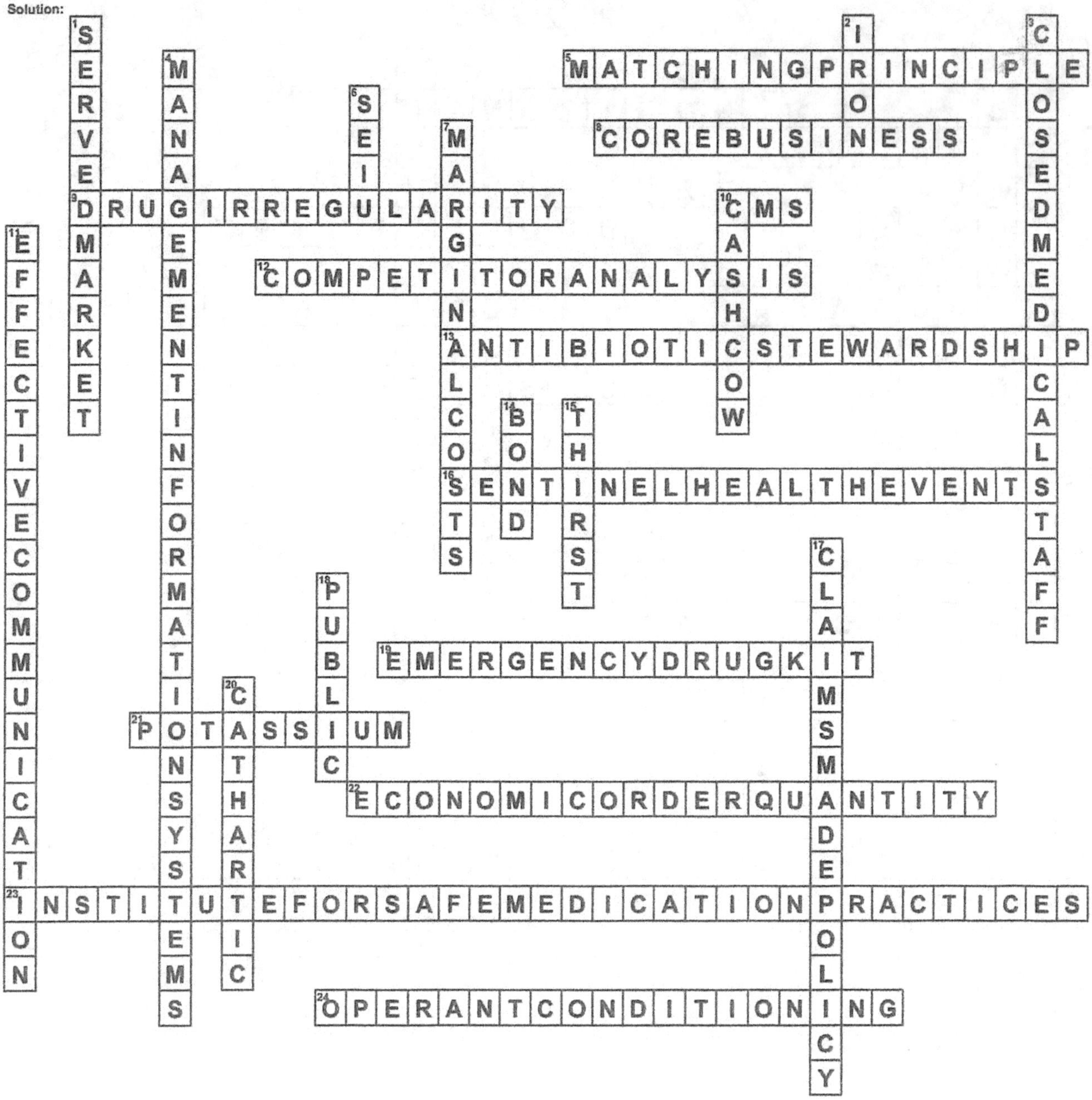

1 SERVEDMARKET
2 IRON
3 CLOSEDMEDICALSTAFF
4 MANAGEMENTINFORMATIONSYSTEMS
5 MATCHINGPRINCIPLE
6 SEI
7 MARGINALCOSTS
8 COREBUSINESS
9 DRUGIRREGULARITY
10 CMS
CASHCOW
11 EFFECTIVECOMMUNICATION
12 COMPETITORANALYSIS
13 ANTIBIOTICSTEWARDSHIP
14 BOND
15 THIRST
16 SENTINELHEALTHEVENTS
17 CLAIMSMADEPOLICY
18 PUBLIC
19 EMERGENCYDRUGKIT
20 CATHARTIC
21 POTASSIUM
22 ECONOMICORDERQUANTITY
23 INSTITUTEFORSAFEMEDICATIONPRACTICES
24 OPERANTCONDITIONING

PUZZLE # 18

Solution:

1 REDBLOODCOUNT
2 HEALTHCAREFRAUD
3 HOMEANDCOMMUNITYBASEDSERVICES
4 RATIOHIRING
5 MEDICALDIRECTOR
6 DISPARATEIMPACT
7 PREVENTIVEMAINTENANCE
8 TWOHUNDREDFORTY
9 RESTORATIVECARE
10 NOTHINGBYMOUTH
11 EFFECTIVECOMMUNICATION
12 DISCRIMINATION
13 SUPPLIER
14 PREGNANCYDISCRIMINATIONACT
15 MAN
16 PSYCHIATRIST
17 SYSTEMSTHEORY
18 LANGUAGEBARRIER
19 RESPITECARE
20 LASTWILLANDTESTAMENT
21 CRIME
22 RESIDENTRIGHTS
23 LEADBYWALKINGAROUND
24 NAIVELISTENING
25 SPECIALSURVEY

PUZZLE # 19

Solution:

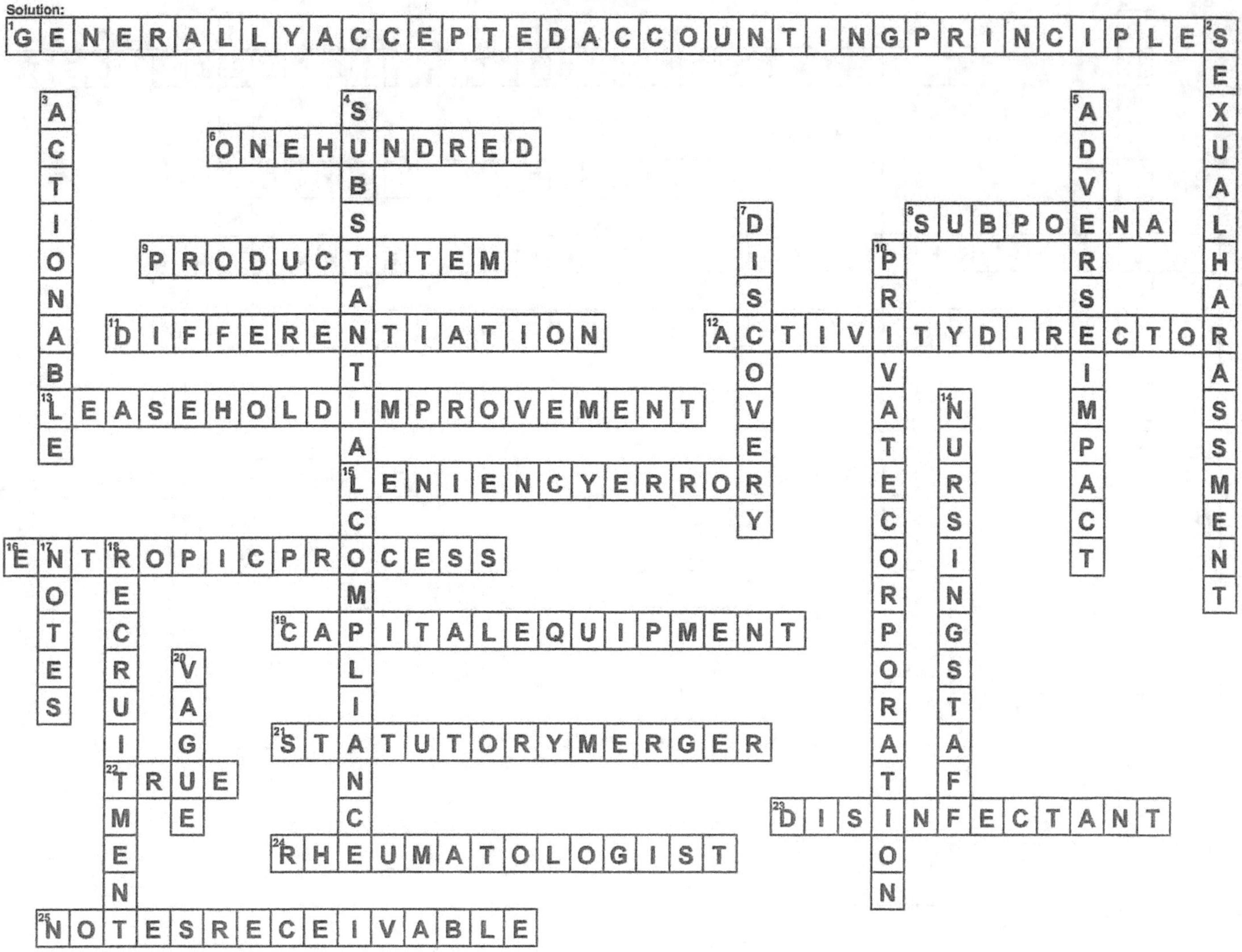

1 GENERALLYACCEPTEDACCOUNTINGPRINCIPLES
2 SEXUALHARASSMENT
3 ACTIONABLE
4 SUBSTANTIALCOMPLIANCE
5 ADVERSEIMPACT
6 ONEHUNDRED
7 DISCOVERY
8 SUBPOENA
9 PRODUCTITEM
10 PRIVATECORPORATION
11 DIFFERENTIATION
12 ACTIVITYDIRECTOR
13 LEASEHOLDIMPROVEMENT
14 NURSINGSTAFF
15 LENIENCYERROR
16 ENTROPICPROCESS
17 NOTES
18 RECRUITMENT
19 CAPITALEQUIPMENT
20 VAGUE
21 STATUTORYMERGER
22 TRUE
23 DISINFECTANT
24 RHEUMATOLOGIST
25 NOTESRECEIVABLE

PUZZLE # 20

Solution:

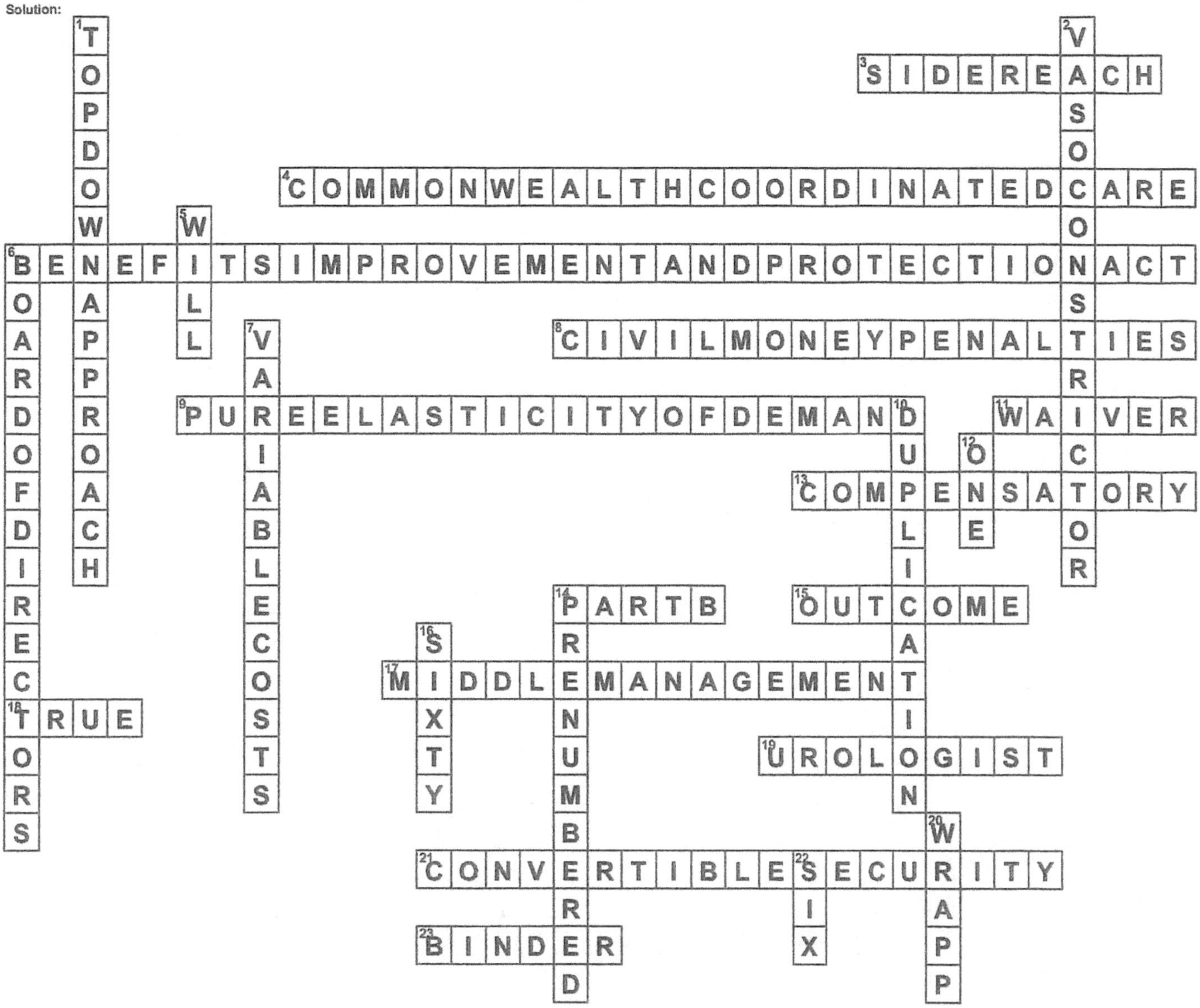
1 TOPDOWNAPPROACH
2 VASOCONSTRICTOR
3 SIDEREACH
4 COMMONWEALTHCOORDINATEDCARE
5 WILL
6 BENEFITSIMPROVEMENTANDPROTECTIONACT
6 BOARDOFDIRECTORS
7 VARIABLECOSTS
8 CIVILMONEYPENALTIES
9 PUREELASTICITYOFDEMAND
10 DUPLICATION
11 WAIVER
12 ONE
13 COMPENSATORY
14 PARTB
14 PRENUMBERED
15 OUTCOME
16 SIXTY
17 MIDDLEMANAGEMENT
18 TRUE
19 UROLOGIST
20 WRAPP
21 CONVERTIBLESECURITY
22 SIX
23 BINDER

PUZZLE # 21

Solution:

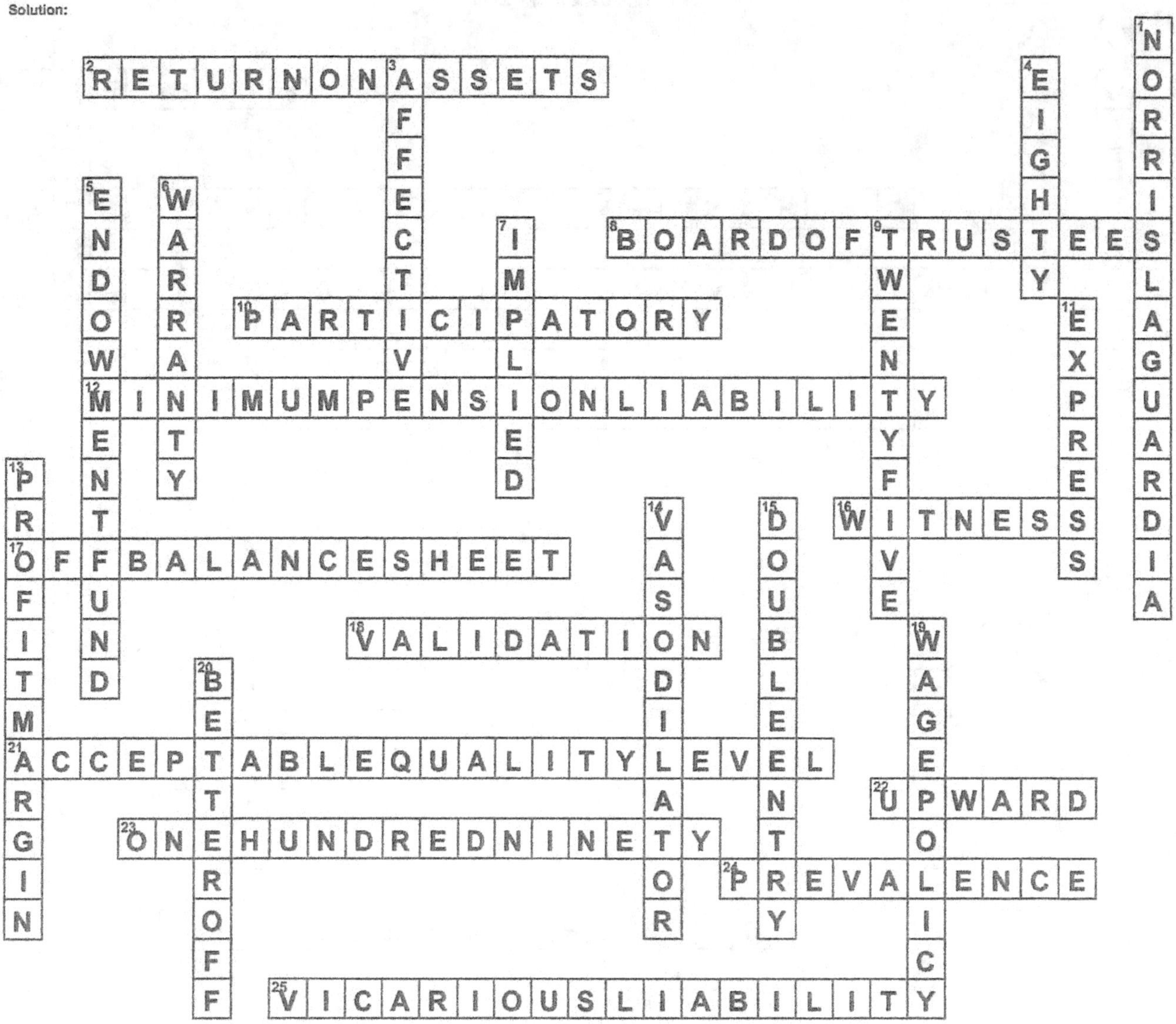
1 NORRISLAGUARDIA
2 RETURNONASSETS
3 AFFECTIVE
4 EIGHTY
5 ENDOWMENTFUND
6 WARRANTY
7 IMPLIED
8 BOARDOFTRUSTEES
9 TWENTYFIVE
10 PARTICIPATORY
11 EXPRESS
12 MINIMUMPENSIONLIABILITY
13 PROFITMARGIN
14 VASODILATOR
15 DOUBLEENTRY
16 WITNESS
17 OFFBALANCESHEET
18 VALIDATION
19 WAGEPOLIC
20 BETTEROFF
21 ACCEPTABLEQUALITYLEVEL
22 UPWARD
23 ONEHUNDREDNINETY
24 PREVALENCE
25 VICARIOUSLIABILITY

PUZZLE # 22

Solution:

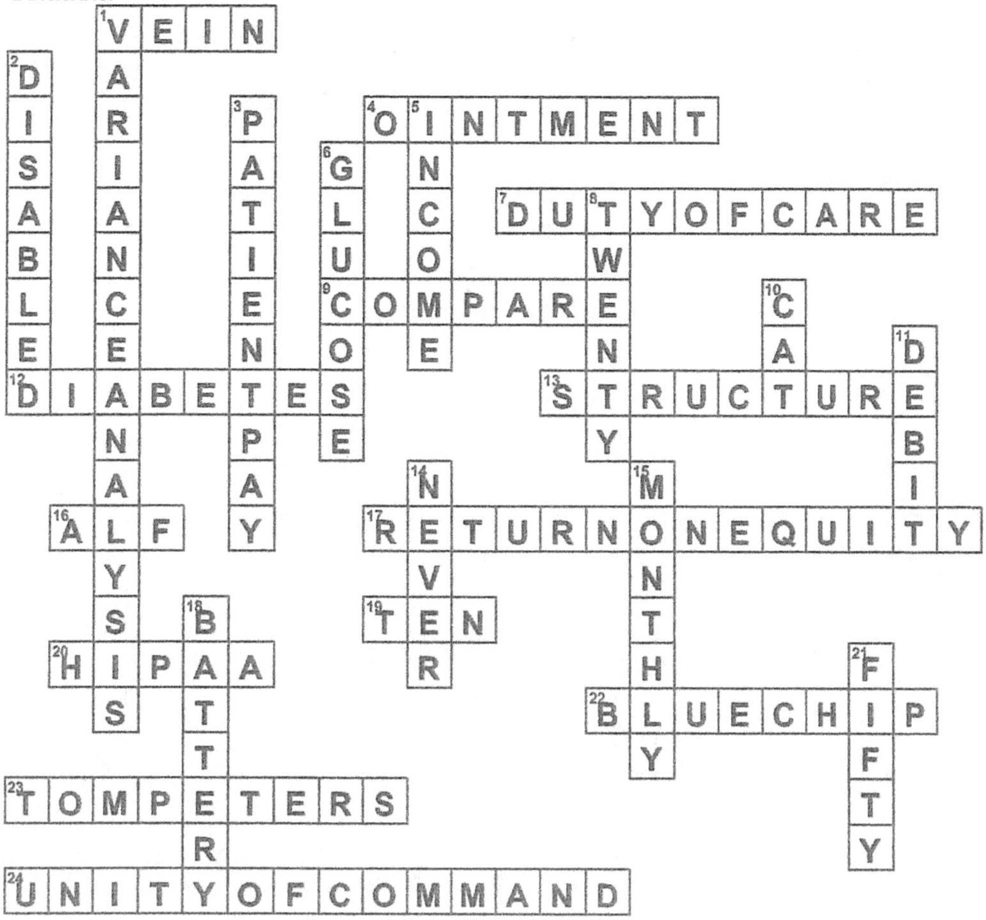
1 VEIN
1 VARIANCEANALYSIS
2 DISABLE
3 PATIENTPAY
4 OINTMENT
5 INCOME
6 GLUCOSE
7 DUTYOFCARE
8 TWENTY
9 COMPARE
10 CA
11 DEBIT
12 DIABETES
13 STRUCTURE
14 NEVER
15 MONTHLY
16 ALF
17 RETURNONEQUITY
18 BATTER
19 TEN
20 HIPAA
21 FIFTY
22 BLUECHIP
23 TOMPETERS
24 UNITYOFCOMMAND

PUZZLE # 23

Solution:

1. CONSTRUCTVALIDITY
2. REIMBURSABLETHERAPYMINUTES
3. ATTENDINGPHYSICIAN
4. ANALYSIS
5. JUSTINTIME
6. JOBENRICHMENT
7. KERRMILLS
8. QUALITYATTHESOURCE
9. RAILWAYLABOR
10. NINETEEN
11. TRUE
12. JOBWORTH
13. ONEHUNDRED
14. KRIEGAL
15. CONSERVATISM
16. JURISDICTION
17. JOBEVALUATION
18. LABORMARKET
19. KIDNEYS
20. COORDINATION
21. ORTHOPEDIST
22. STATEMENTOFCHANGES
23. NINJASOFJOY
24. MATERIALITY
25. CASHEQUIVALENT

PUZZLE # 24

Solution:

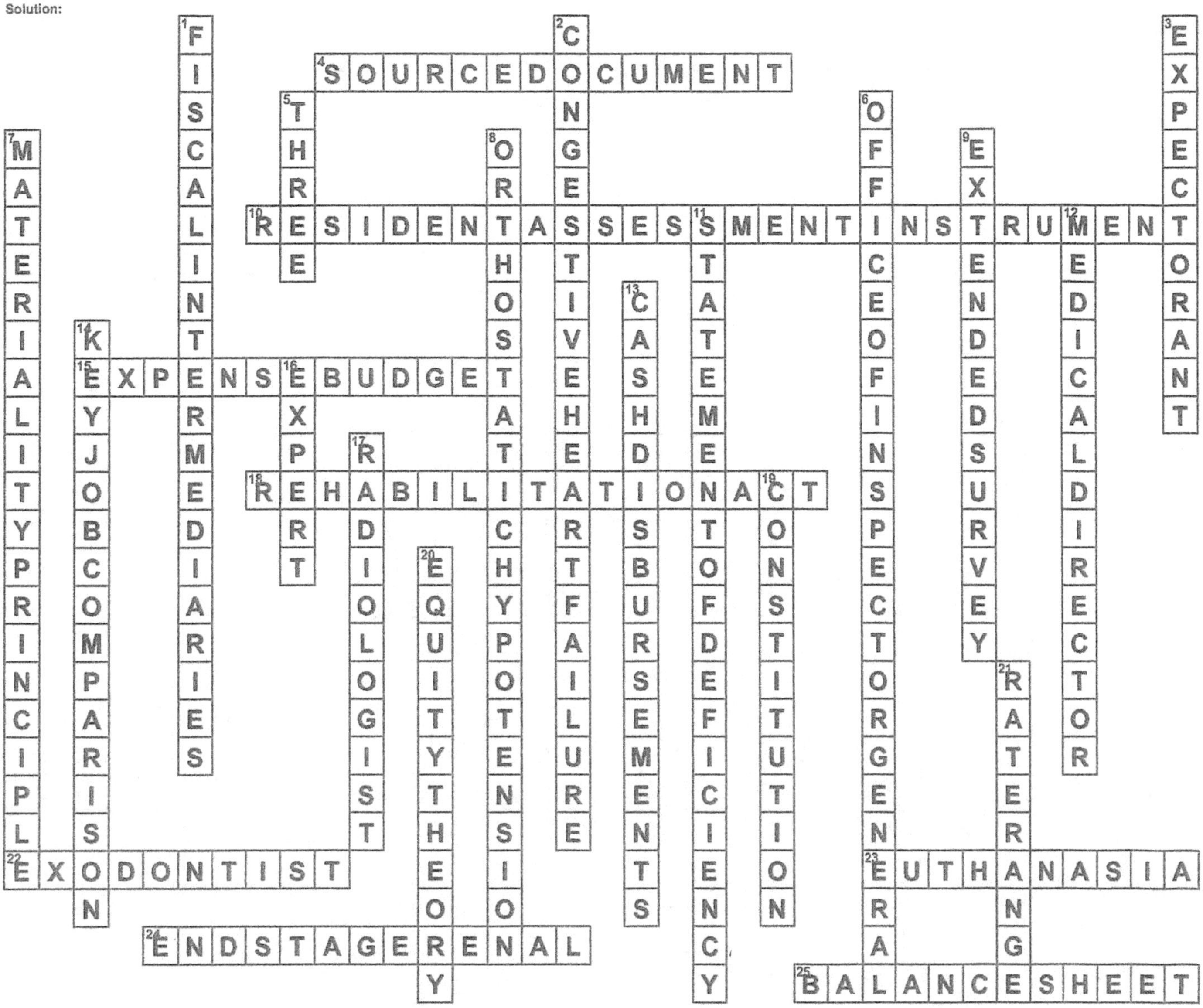

1 FISCALINTERMEDIARIES
2 CONGESTIVEHEARTFAILURE
3 EXPECTORANT
4 SOURCEDOCUMENT
5 THREE
6 OFFICEOFINSPECTORGENERA
7 MATERIALITYPRINCIPL
8 ORTHOSTATICHYPOTENSIO
9 EXTENDEDSURVEY
10 RESIDENTASSESSMENTINSTRUMENT
11 STATEMENTOFDEFICIENCY
12 MEDICALDIRECTOR
13 CASHDISBURSEMENTS
14 KEYJOBCOMPARISON
15 EXPENSEBUDGET
16 EXPERT
17 RADIOLOGIST
18 REHABILITATIONACT
19 CONSTITUTION
20 EQUITYTHEORY
21 RATERRANG
22 EXODONTIST
23 EUTHANASIA
24 ENDSTAGERENAL
25 BALANCESHEET

PUZZLE # 25

Solution:

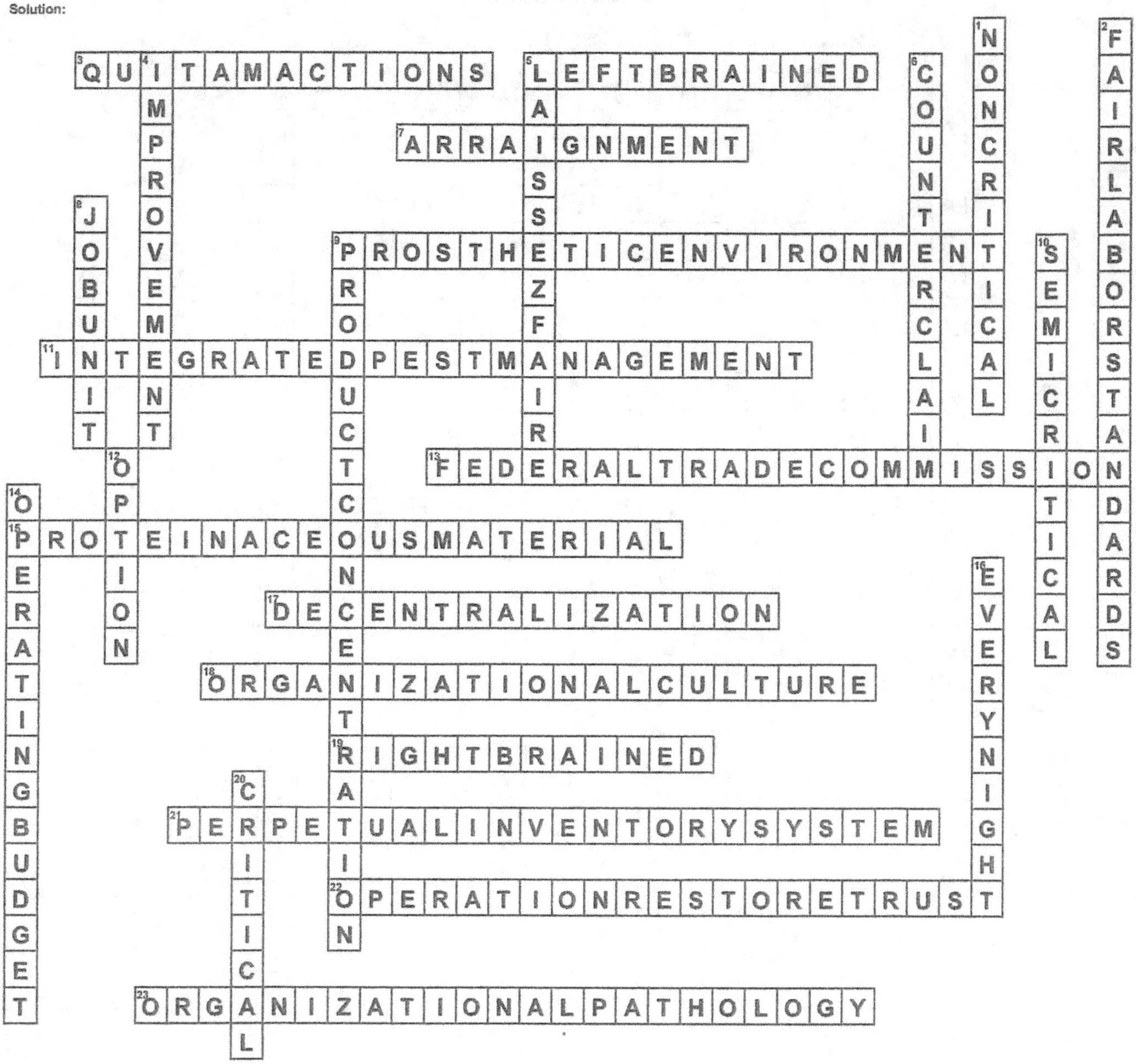

1 NONCRITICAL
2 FAIRLABORSTANDARDS
3 QUITAMACTIONS
4 IMPROVEMENT
5 LEFTBRAINED
5 LAISSEZFAIR
6 COUNTERCLAIM
7 ARRAIGNMENT
8 JOBUNIT
9 PROSTHETICENVIRONMENT
9 PRODUCTCONCENTRATION
10 SEMICRITICAL
11 INTEGRATEDPESTMANAGEMENT
12 OPTION
13 FEDERALTRADECOMMISSION
14 OPERATINGBUDGET
15 PROTEINACEOUSMATERIAL
16 EVERYNIGHT
17 DECENTRALIZATION
18 ORGANIZATIONALCULTURE
19 RIGHTBRAINED
20 CRITICAL
21 PERPETUALINVENTORYSYSTEM
22 OPERATIONRESTORETRUST
23 ORGANIZATIONALPATHOLOGY

PUZZLE # 26

Solution:

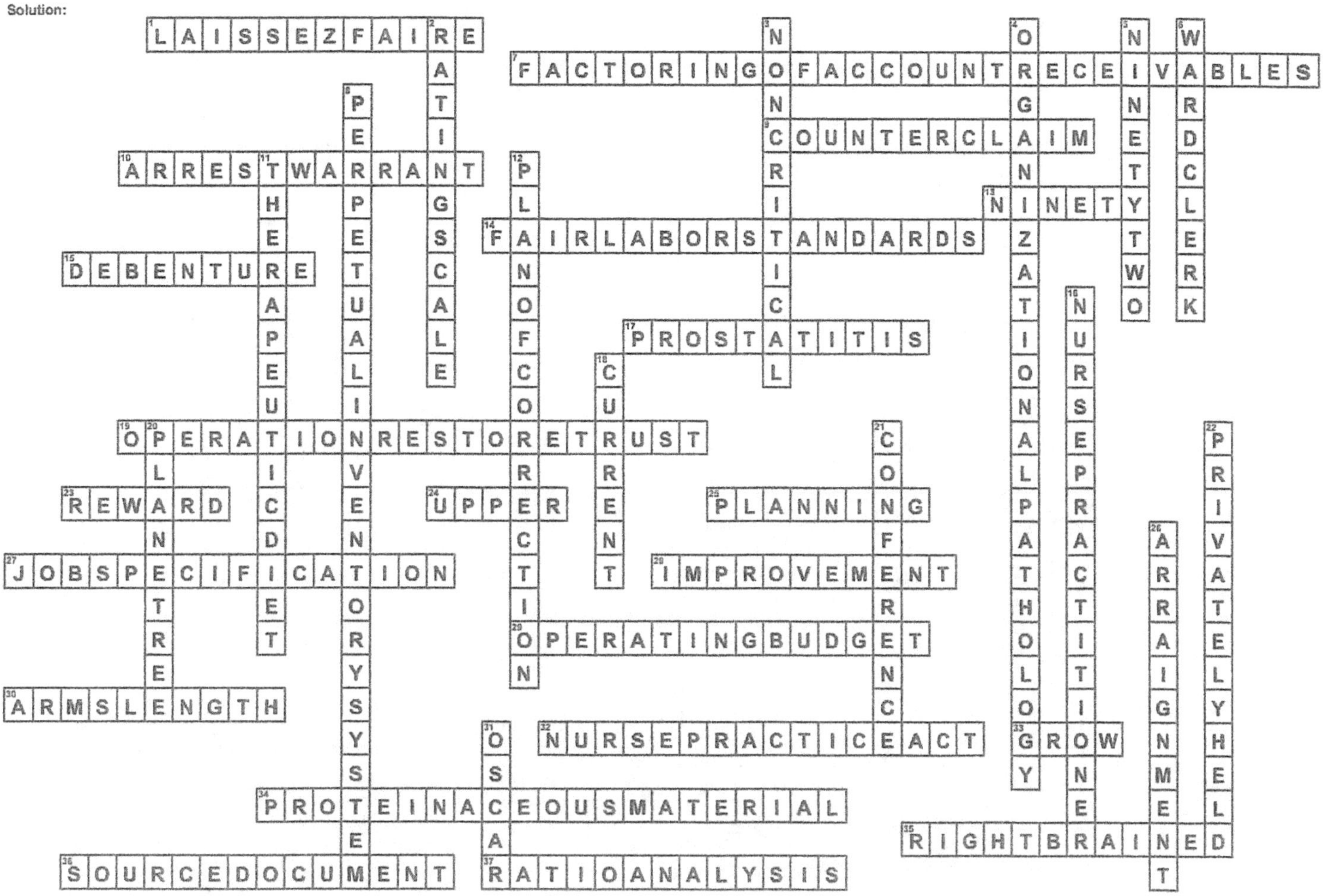

1 LAISSEZFAIRE
2 RATINGSCALE
3 NONCRITICAL
4 ORGANIZATIONALPATHOLOGY
5 NINETYTWO
6 WORDCLERK
7 FACTORINGOFACCOUNTRECEIVABLES
8 PERPETUALINVENTORYSYSTEM
9 COUNTERCLAIM
10 ARRESTWARRANT
11 THERAPEUTICDIET
12 PLANOFCORRECTION
13 NINETY
14 FAIRLABORSTANDARDS
15 DEBENTURE
16 NURSEPRACTITIONER
17 PROSTATITIS
18 CURRENT
19 OPERATIONRESTORETRUST
20 PLANETREE
21 CONFERENCE
22 PRIVATELYHELD
23 REWARD
24 UPPER
25 PLANNING
26 ARRAIGNMENT
27 JOBSPECIFICATION
28 IMPROVEMENT
29 OPERATINGBUDGET
30 ARMSLENGTH
31 OSCAR
32 NURSEPRACTICEACT
33 GROW
34 PROTEINACEOUSMATERIAL
35 RIGHTBRAINED
36 SOURCEDOCUMENT
37 RATIOANALYSIS

PUZZLE # 27

Solution:

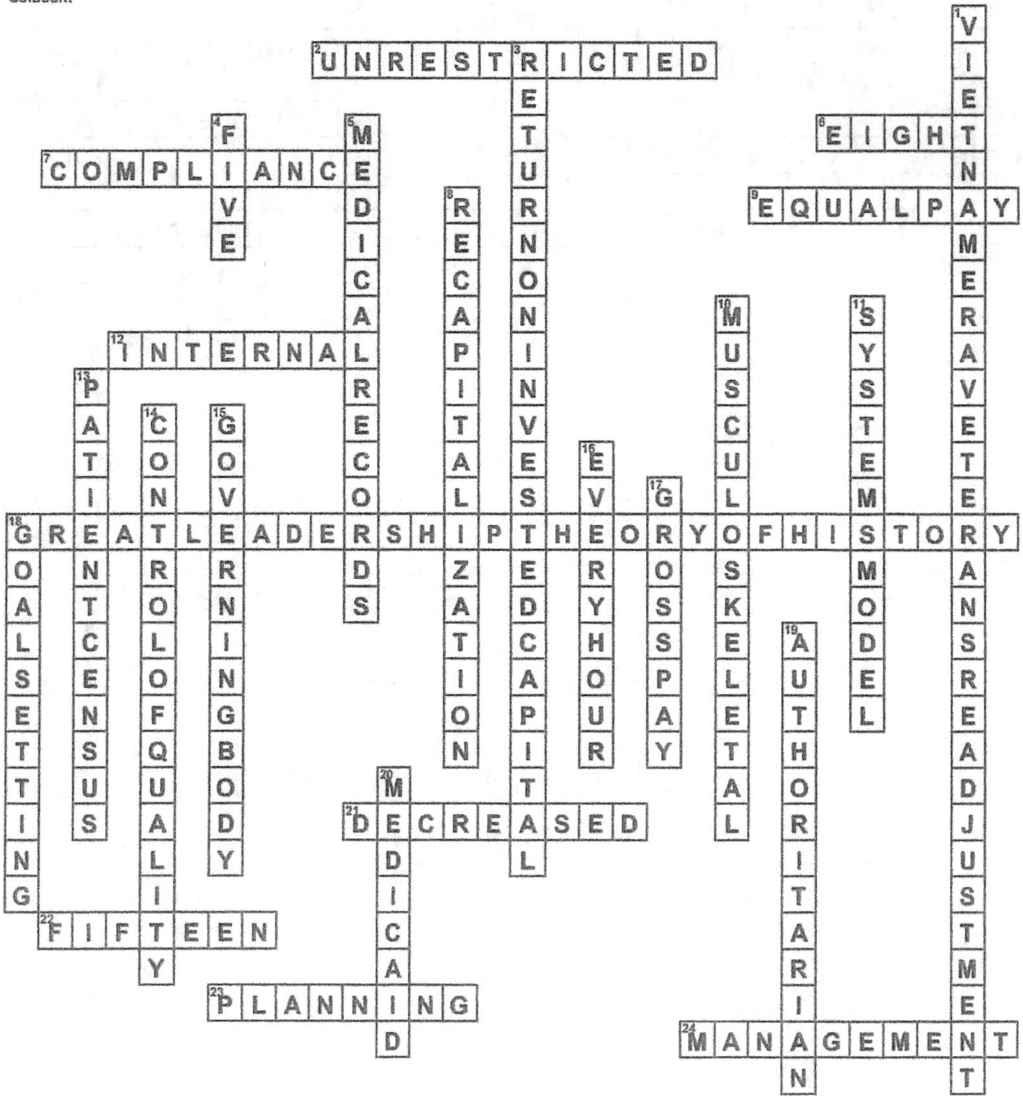

1 VIETNAMERAVETERANSREADJUSTMENT
2 UNRESTRICTED
3 RETURNONINVESTEDCAPITAL
4 FIVE
5 MEDICALRECORDS
6 EIGHT
7 COMPLIANCE
8 RECAPITALIZATION
9 EQUALPAY
10 MUSCULOSKELETAL
11 SYSTEMMODEL
12 INTERNAL
13 PATIENTCENSUS
14 CONTROLOFQUALITY
15 GOVERNINGBODY
16 EVERYHOUR
17 GOSSPAY
18 GREATLEADERSHIPTHEORYOFHISTORY
18 GOALSETTING
19 AUTHORITARIAN
20 MEDICAID
21 DECREASED
22 FIFTEEN
23 PLANNING
24 MANAGEMENT

PUZZLE # 28

Solution:

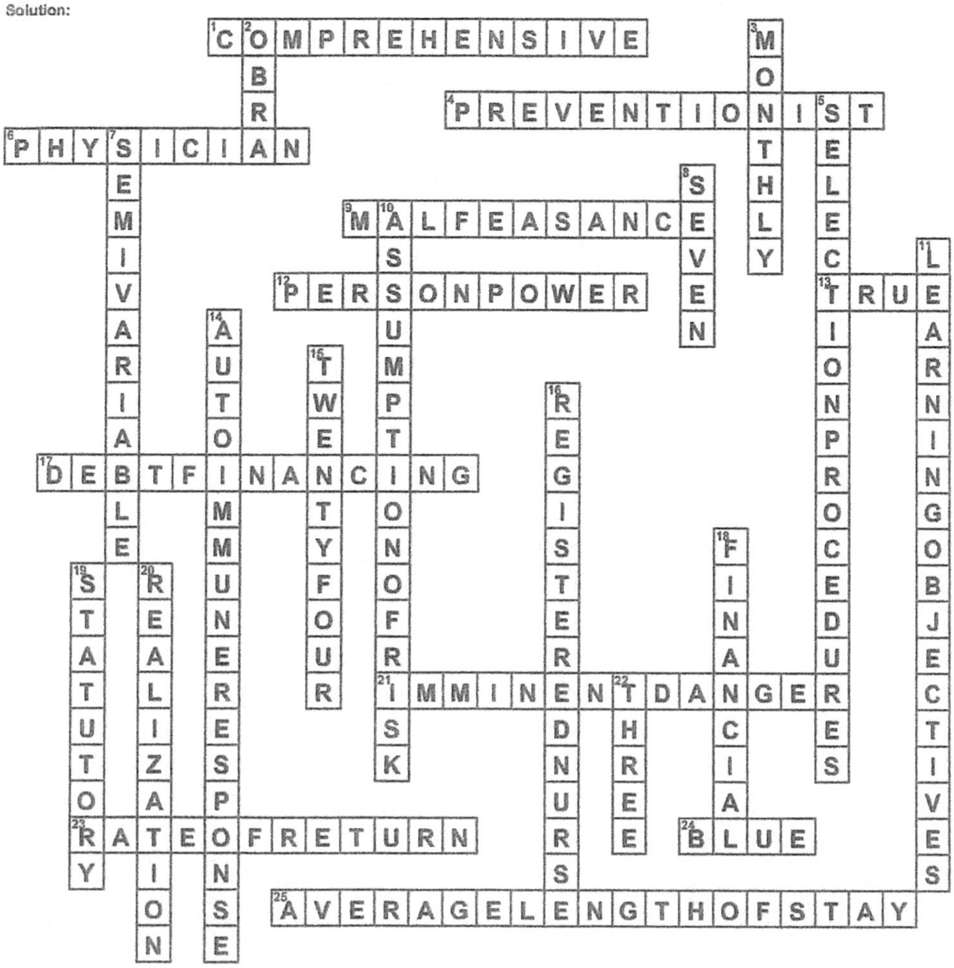

1 COMPREHENSIVE
2 OBRA
3 MONTHLY
4 PREVENTIONIST
5 SELECTIONPROCEDURES
6 PHYSICIAN
7 SEMIVARIABLE
8 SEVEN
9 MALFEASANCE
10 ASSUMPTIONOFRISK
11 LEARNINGOBJECTIVES
12 PERSONPOWER
13 TRUE
14 AUTOIMMUNERESPONSE
15 TWENTYFOUR
16 REGISTEREDNURSES
17 DEBTFINANCING
18 FINANCIAL
19 STATUTORY
20 REALIZATION
21 IMMINENTDANGER
22 THREE
23 RATEOFRETURN
24 BLUE
25 AVERAGELENGTHOFSTAY

PUZZLE # 29

Solution:

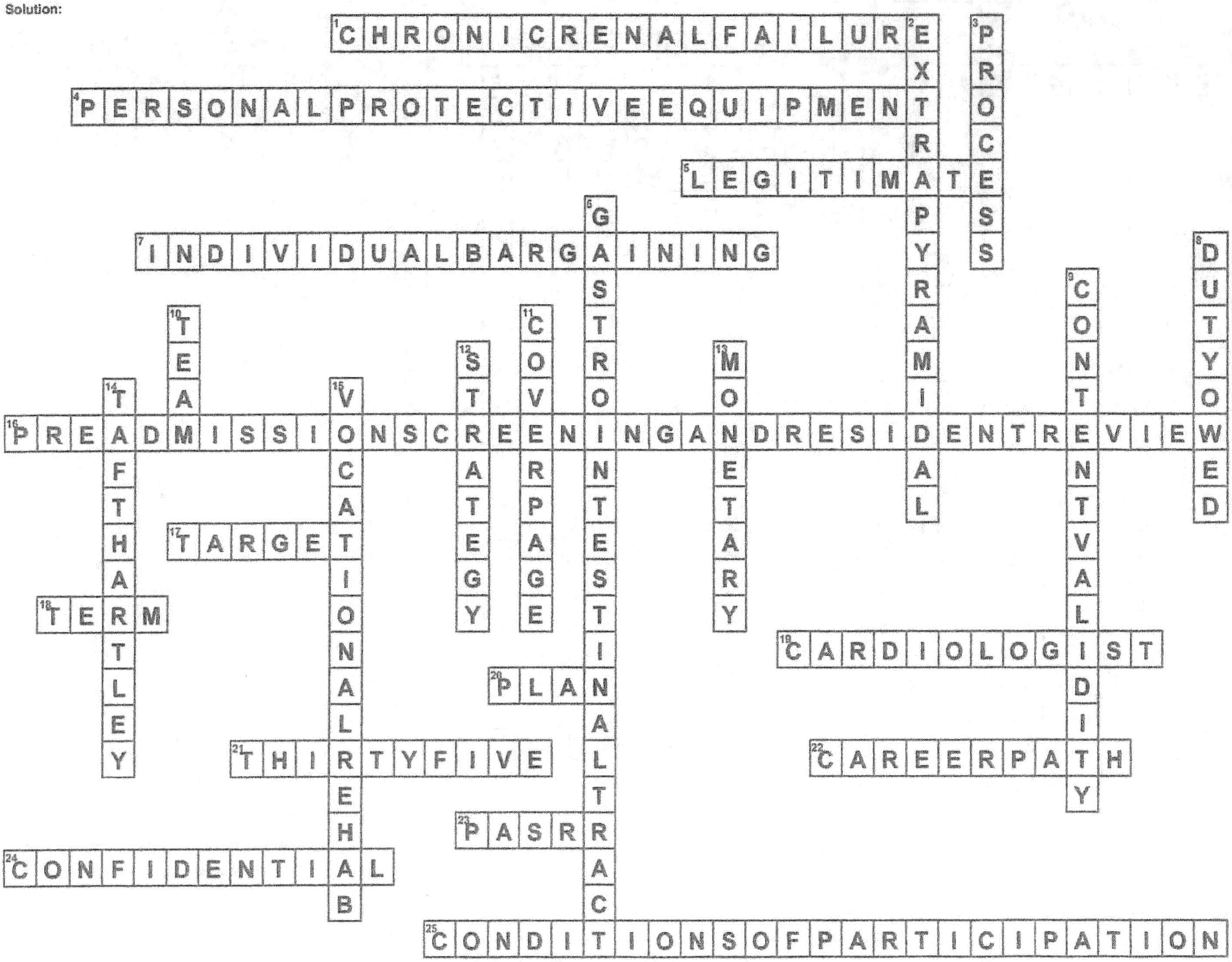

1 CHRONICRENALFAILURE
2 EXTRAPYRAMIDAL
3 PROCESS
4 PERSONALPROTECTIVEEQUIPMENT
5 LEGITIMATE
6 GASTROINTESTINALTRACT
7 INDIVIDUALBARGAINING
8 DUTYOWED
9 CONTENTVALIDITY
10 TEAM
11 COVERPAGE
12 STRATEGY
13 MONETARY
14 TAFTHARTLEY
15 VOCATIONALREHAB
16 PREADMISSIONSCREENINGANDRESIDENTREVIEW
17 TARGET
18 TERM
19 CARDIOLOGIST
20 PLAN
21 THIRTYFIVE
22 CAREERPATH
23 PASRR
24 CONFIDENTIAL
25 CONDITIONSOFPARTICIPATION

PUZZLE # 30

Solution:

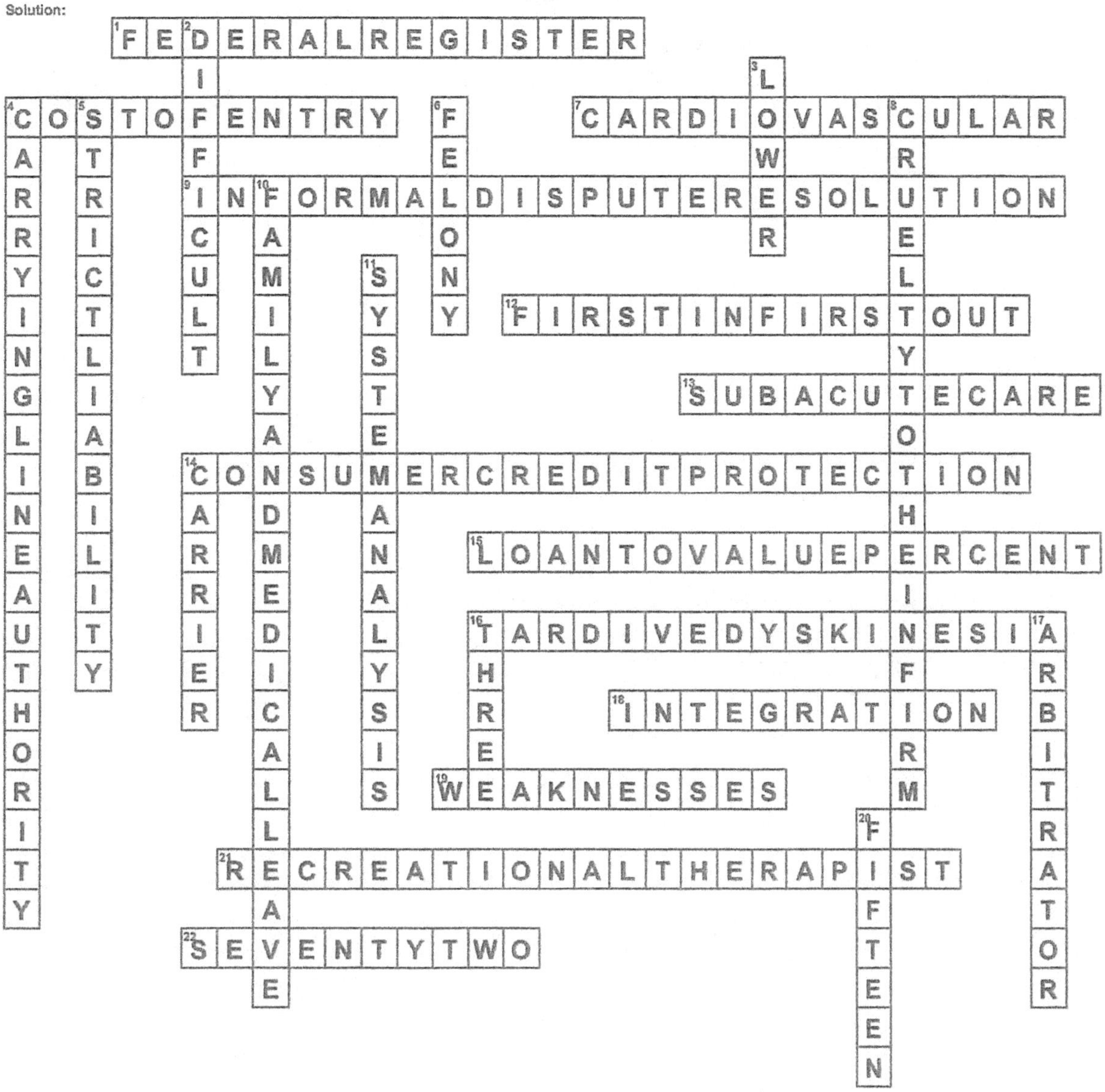
1 FEDERALREGISTER
2 DIFFICULT
3 LOWER
4 COSTOFENTRY
4 CARRYINGLINEAUTHORITY
5 STRICTLIABILITY
6 FELONY
7 CARDIOVASCULAR
8 CRUELTYTOTHEINFIRM
9 INFORMALDISPUTERESOLUTION
10 FAMILYANDMEDICALLEAVE
11 SYSTEMSANALYSIS
12 FIRSTINFIRSTOUT
13 SUBACUTECARE
14 CONSUMERCREDITPROTECTION
14 CARRIER
15 LOANTOVALUEPERCENT
16 TARDIVEDYSKINESIA
16 THREE
17 ARBITRATOR
18 INTEGRATION
19 WEAKNESSES
20 FIFTEEN
21 RECREATIONALTHERAPIST
22 SEVENTYTWO

PUZZLE # 31

Solution:

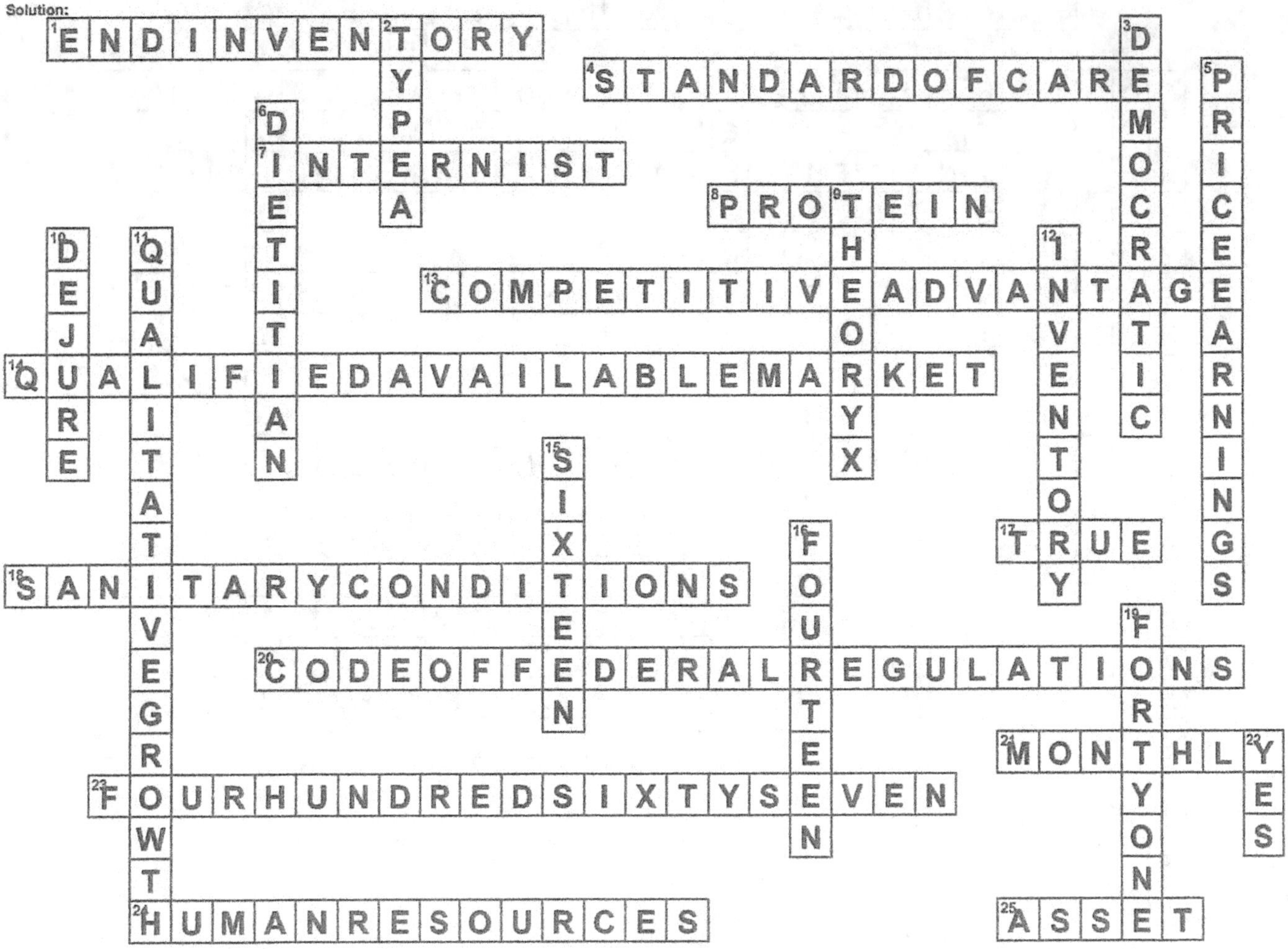

1 ENDINVENTORY
2 TYPEA
3 DEMOCRATIC
4 STANDARDOFCARE
5 PRICEEARNINGS
6 DIETITIAN
7 INTERNIST
8 PROTEIN
9 THEORYX
10 DEJURE
11 QUALITATIVEGROWTH
12 INVENTORY
13 COMPETITIVEADVANTAGE
14 QUALIFIEDAVAILABLEMARKET
15 SIXTEEN
16 FOURTEEN
17 TRUE
18 SANITARYCONDITIONS
19 FORTYONE
20 CODEOFFEDERALREGULATIONS
21 MONTHLY
22 YES
23 FOURHUNDREDSIXTYSEVEN
24 HUMANRESOURCES
25 ASSET

PUZZLE # 32

Solution:

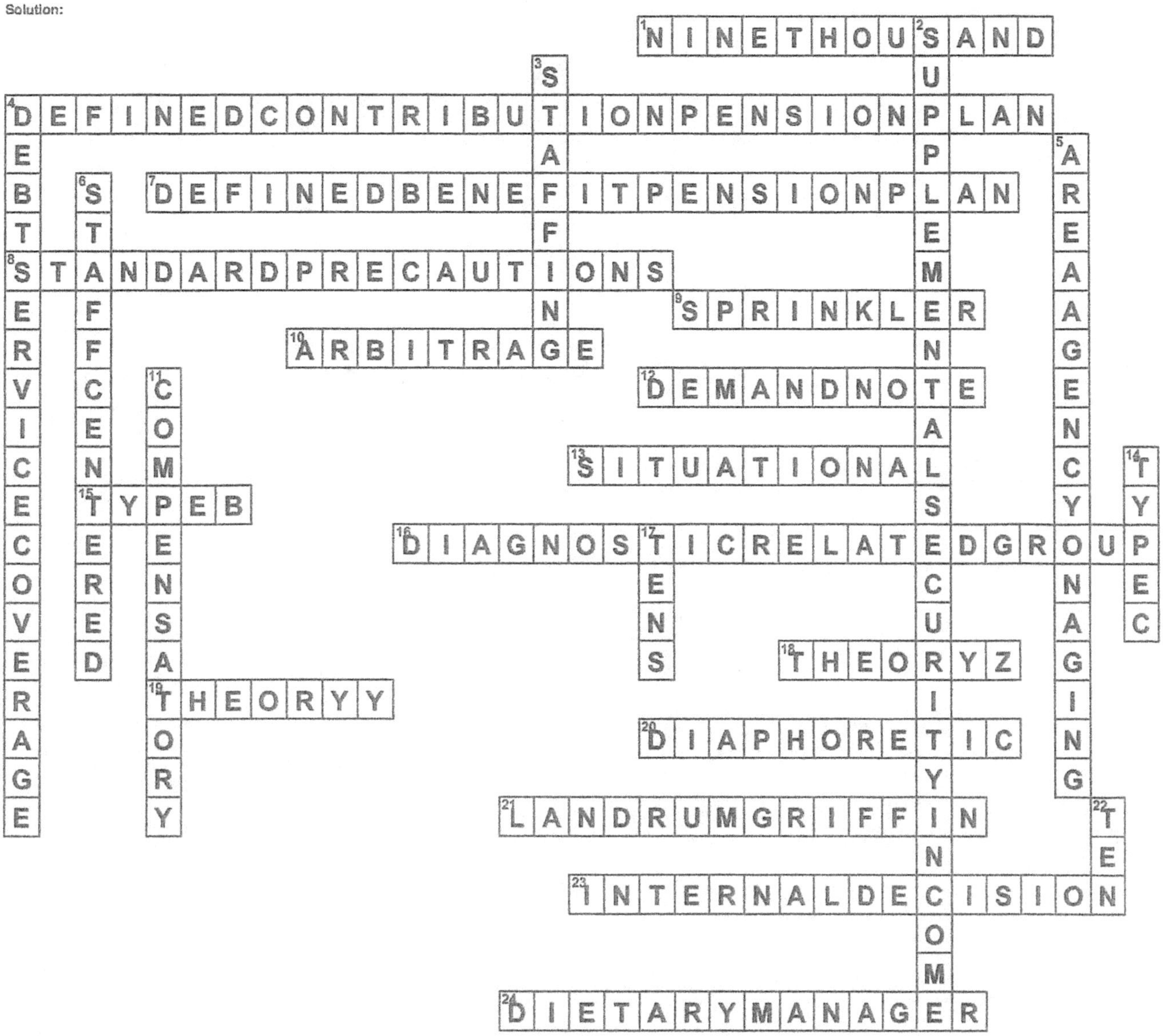

1 NINETHOUSAND
2 SUPPLEMENTALSECURITYINCOME
3 STAFFING
4 DEFINEDCONTRIBUTIONPENSIONPLAN
4 DEBTSERVICECOVERAGE
5 AREAAGENCYONAGING
6 STAFFCENTERED
7 DEFINEDBENEFITPENSIONPLAN
8 STANDARDPRECAUTIONS
9 SPRINKLER
10 ARBITRAGE
11 COMPENSATORY
12 DEMANDNOTE
13 SITUATIONAL
14 TYPEC
15 TYPEB
16 DIAGNOSTICRELATEDGROUP
17 TENS
18 THEORYZ
19 THEORYY
20 DIAPHORETIC
21 LANDRUMGRIFFIN
22 TEN
23 INTERNALDECISION
24 DIETARYMANAGER

PUZZLE # 33

Solution:

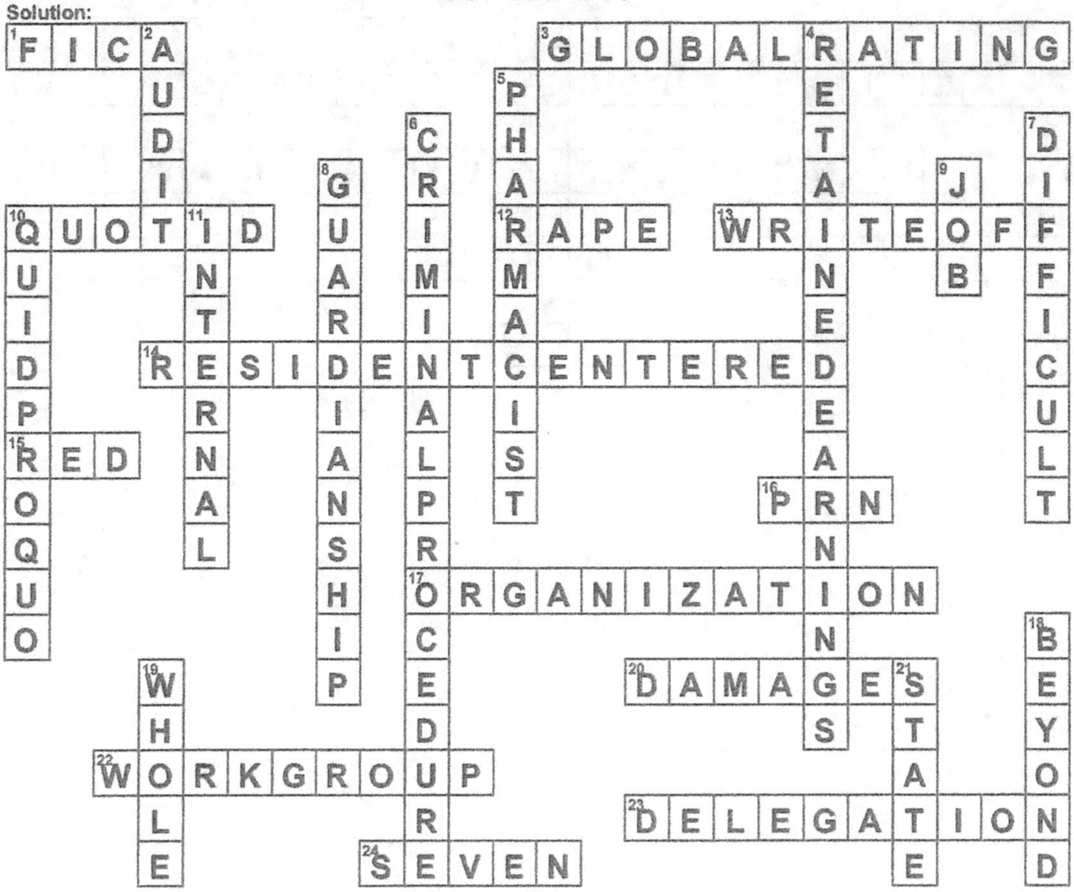
1 FICA
2 AUDIT
3 GLOBALRATING
4 RETAINEDEARNINGS
5 PHARMACIST
6 CRIMINALPROCEDURE
7 DIFFICULT
8 GUARDIANSHIP
9 JOB
10 QUOTID
10 QUIDPROQUO
11 INTERNAL
12 RAPE
13 WRITEOFF
14 RESIDENTCENTERED
15 RED
16 PRN
17 ORGANIZATION
18 BEYOND
19 WHOLE
20 DAMAGES
21 STATE
22 WORKGROUP
23 DELEGATION
24 SEVEN

PUZZLE # 34

Solution:

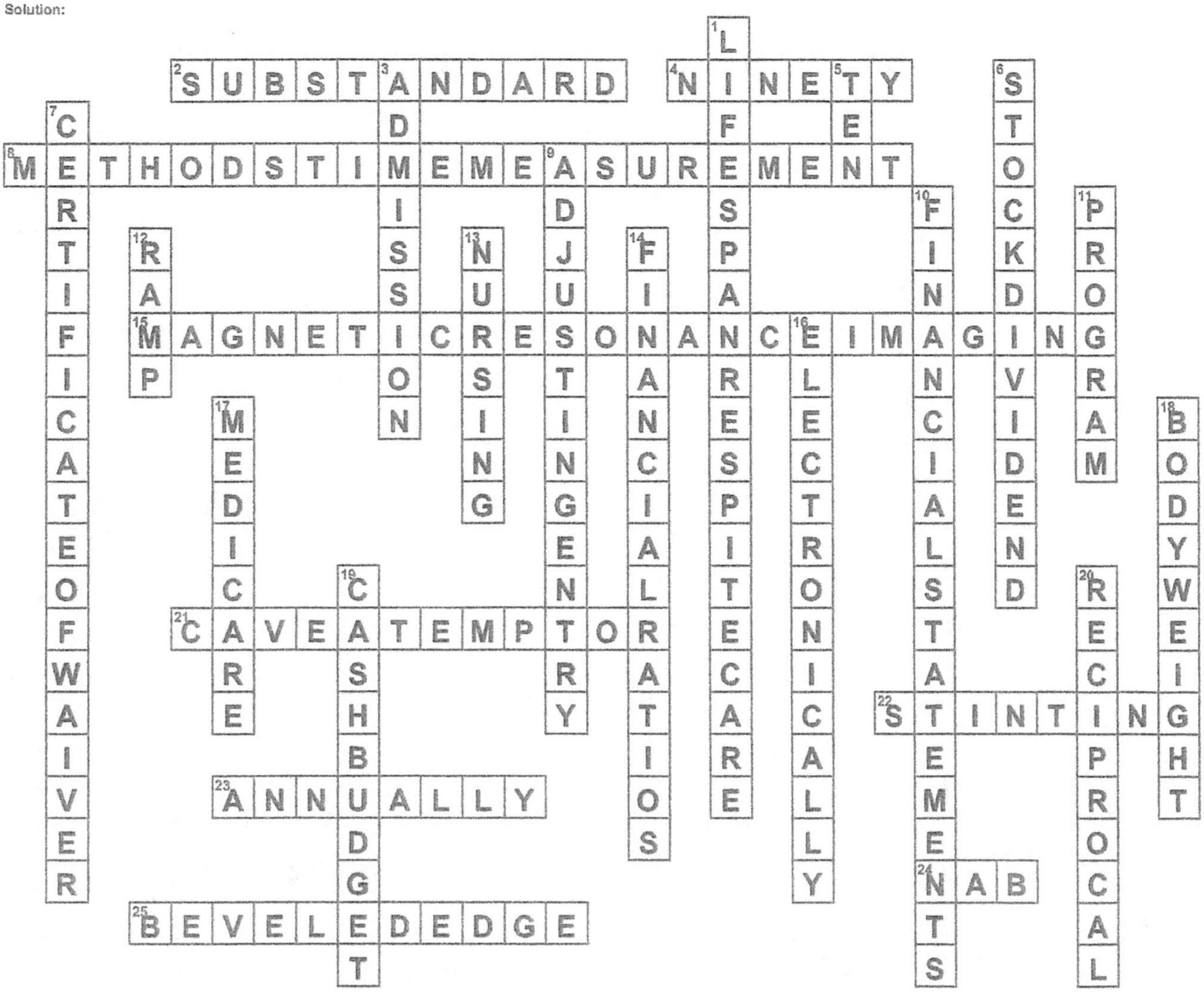

1 LIFESPANRESPITECARE
2 SUBSTANDARD
3 ADMISSION
4 NINETY
5 TEN
6 STOCKDIVIDEND
7 CERTIFICATEOFWAIVER
8 METHODSTIMEMEASUREMENT
9 ADJUSTINGENTRY
10 FINANCIALSTATEMENTS
11 PROGRAM
12 RAMP
13 NURSING
14 FINANCIALRATIOS
15 MAGNETICRESONANCEIMAGING
16 ELECTRONICALLY
17 MEDICARE
18 BODYWEIGHT
19 CASHBUDGET
20 RECIPROCAL
21 CAVEATEMPTOR
22 STINTING
23 ANNUALLY
24 NAB
25 BEVELEDEDGE

PUZZLE # 35

Solution:

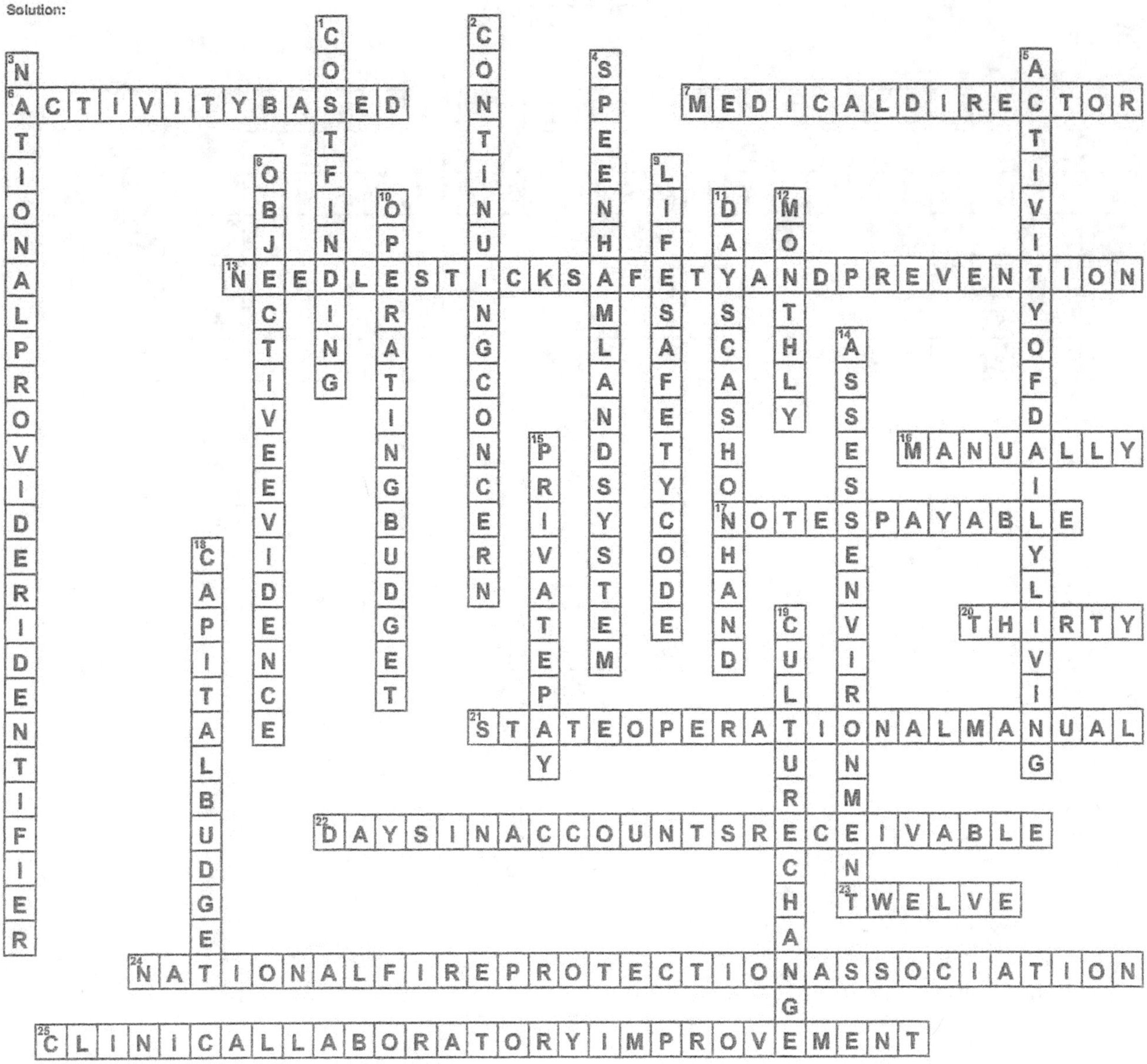
1 COSTFINDING
2 CONTINUINGCONCERN
3 NATIONALPROVIDERIDENTIFIER
4 SPEENHAMLANDSYSTEM
5 ACTIVITYOFDAILYLIVING
6 ACTIVITYBASED
7 MEDICALDIRECTOR
8 OBJECTIVEEVIDENCE
9 LIFESAFETYCODE
10 OPERATINGBUDGET
11 DAYSCASHONHAND
12 MONTHLY
13 NEEDLESTICKSAFETYANDPREVENTION
14 ASSESSENVIRONMENT
15 PRIVATEPAY
16 MANUALLY
17 NOTESPAYABLE
18 CAPITALBUDGET
19 CULTURECHANGE
20 THIRTY
21 STATEOPERATIONALMANUAL
22 DAYSINACCOUNTSRECEIVABLE
23 TWELVE
24 NATIONALFIREPROTECTIONASSOCIATION
25 CLINICALLABORATORYIMPROVEMENT

PUZZLE # 36

Solution:

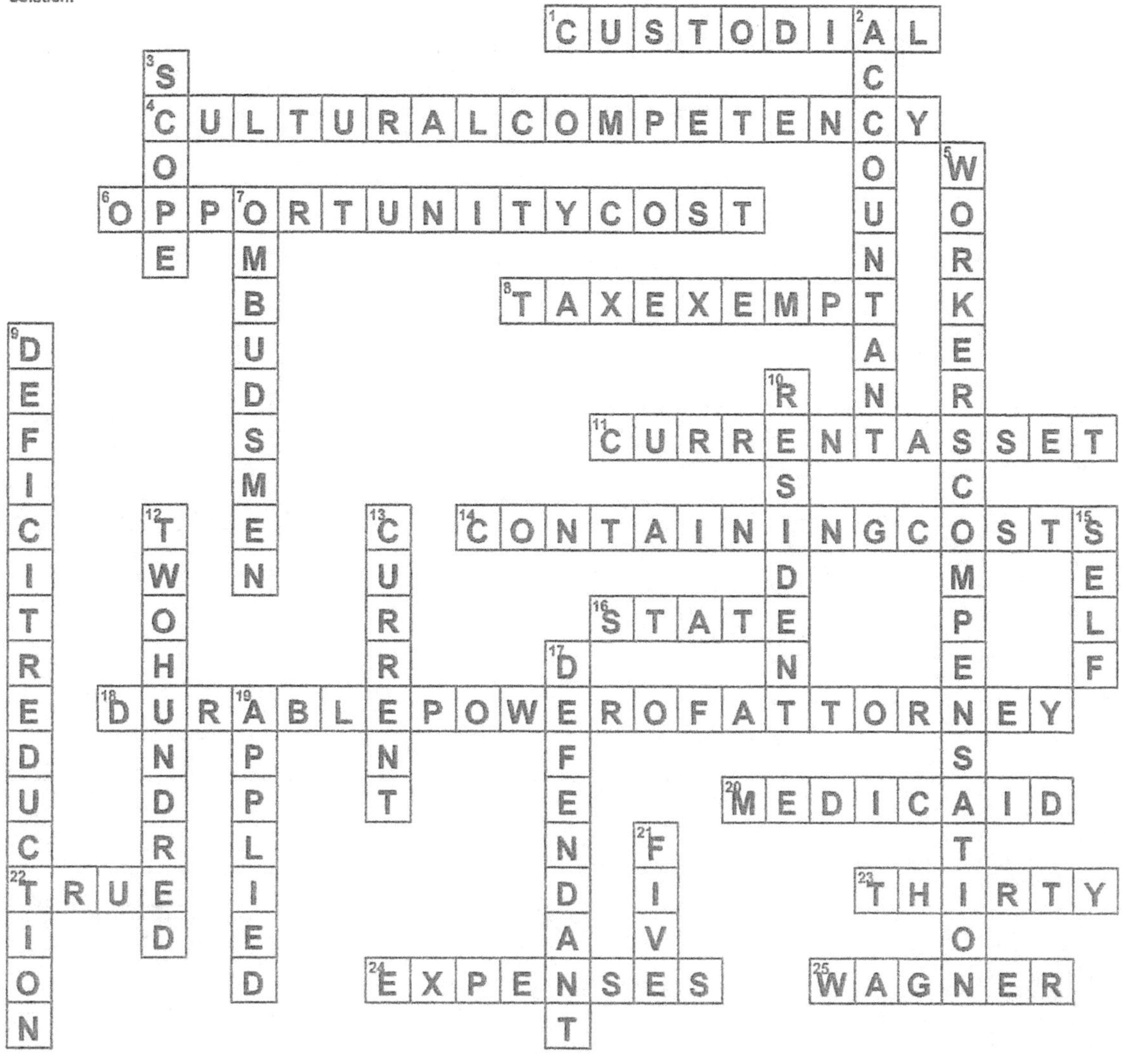

1 CUSTODIAL
2 ACCOUNTANT
3 SCOPE
4 CULTURALCOMPETENCY
5 WORKERSCOMPENSATION
6 OPPORTUNITYCOST
7 OMBUDSMEN
8 TAXEXEMPT
9 DEFICITREDUCTION
10 RESIDENT
11 CURRENTASSET
12 TWOHUNDRED
13 CURRENT
14 CONTAININGCOSTS
15 SELF
16 STATE
17 DEFENDANT
18 DURABLEPOWEROFATTORNEY
19 APPLIED
20 MEDICAID
21 FIVE
22 TRUE
23 THIRTY
24 EXPENSES
25 WAGNER

PUZZLE # 37

Solution:

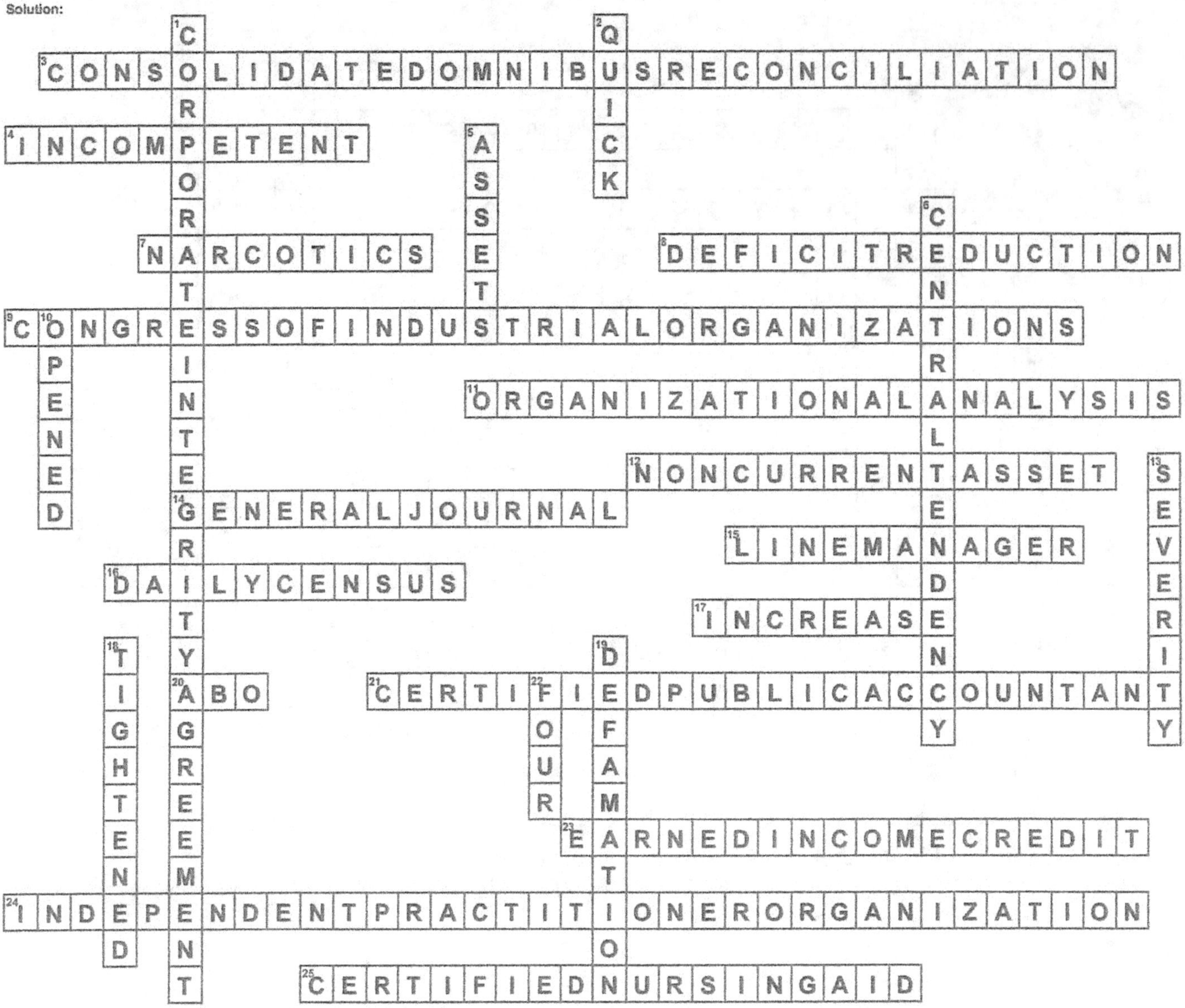

1 CORPORATEINTEGRITYAGREEMENT
2 QUICK
3 CONSOLIDATEDOMNIBUSRECONCILIATION
4 INCOMPETENT
5 ASSETS
6 CENTRALTENDENCY
7 NARCOTICS
8 DEFICITREDUCTION
9 CONGRESSOFINDUSTRIALORGANIZATIONS
10 OPENED
11 ORGANIZATIONALANALYSIS
12 NONCURRENTASSET
13 SEVERITY
14 GENERALJOURNAL
15 LINEMANAGER
16 DAILYCENSUS
17 INCREASE
18 TIGHTENED
19 DEFAMATION
20 ABO
21 CERTIFIEDPUBLICACCOUNTANT
22 FOUR
23 EARNEDINCOMECREDIT
24 INDEPENDENTPRACTITIONERORGANIZATION
25 CERTIFIEDNURSINGAID

PUZZLE # 38

Solution:

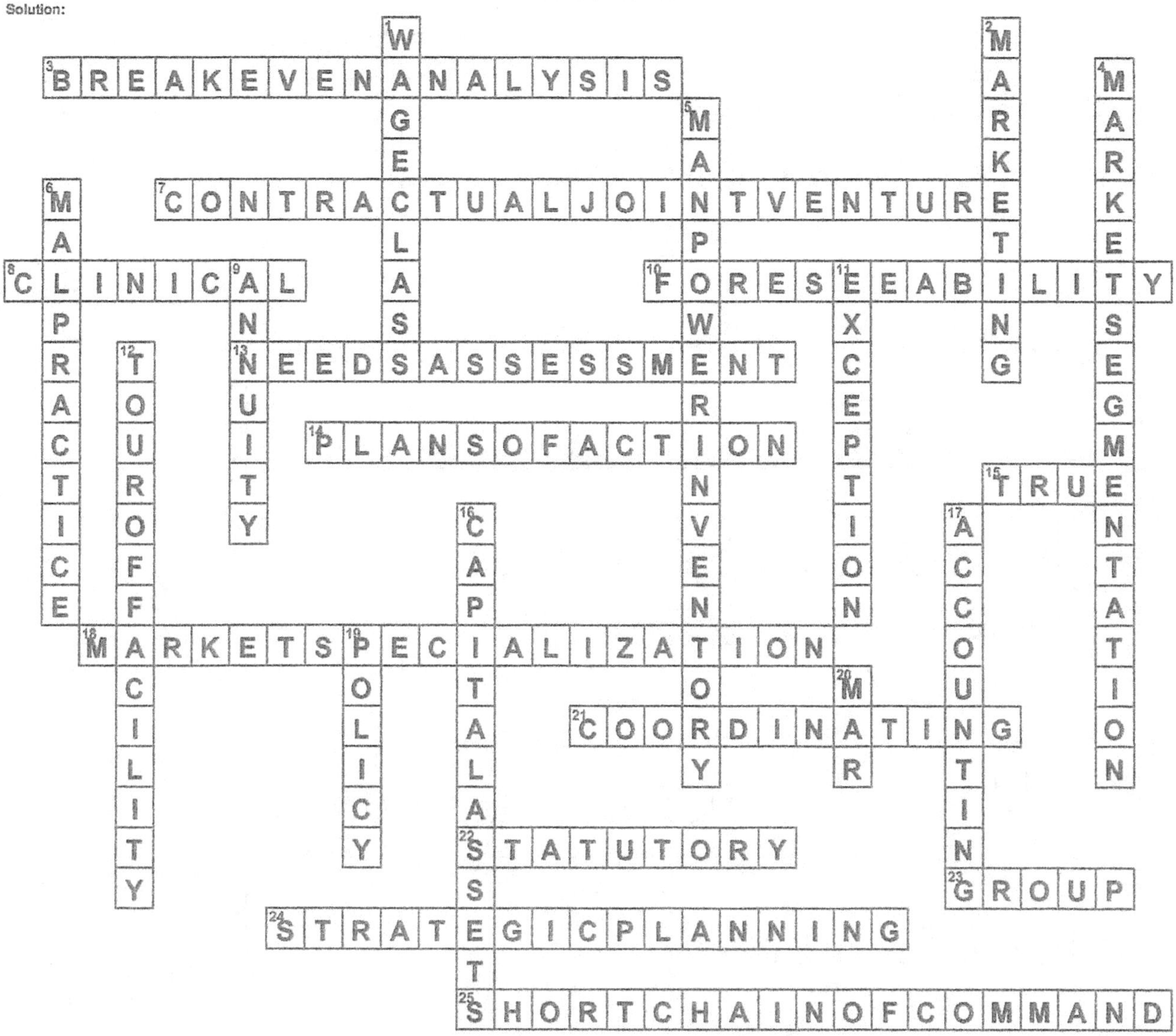

1 WAGECLASS
2 MARKETING
3 BREAKEVENANALYSIS
4 MARKETSEGMENTATION
5 MANPOWERINVENTORY
6 MALPRACTICE
7 CONTRACTUALJOINTVENTURE
8 CLINICAL
9 ANNUITY
10 FORESEEABILITY
11 EXCEPTION
12 TOUROFFACILITY
13 NEEDSASSESSMENT
14 PLANSOFACTION
15 TRUE
16 CAPITALASSETS
17 ACCOUNTING
18 MARKETSPECIALIZATION
19 POLICY
20 MAR
21 COORDINATING
22 STATUTORY
23 GROUP
24 STRATEGICPLANNING
25 SHORTCHAINOFCOMMAND

PUZZLE # 39

Solution:

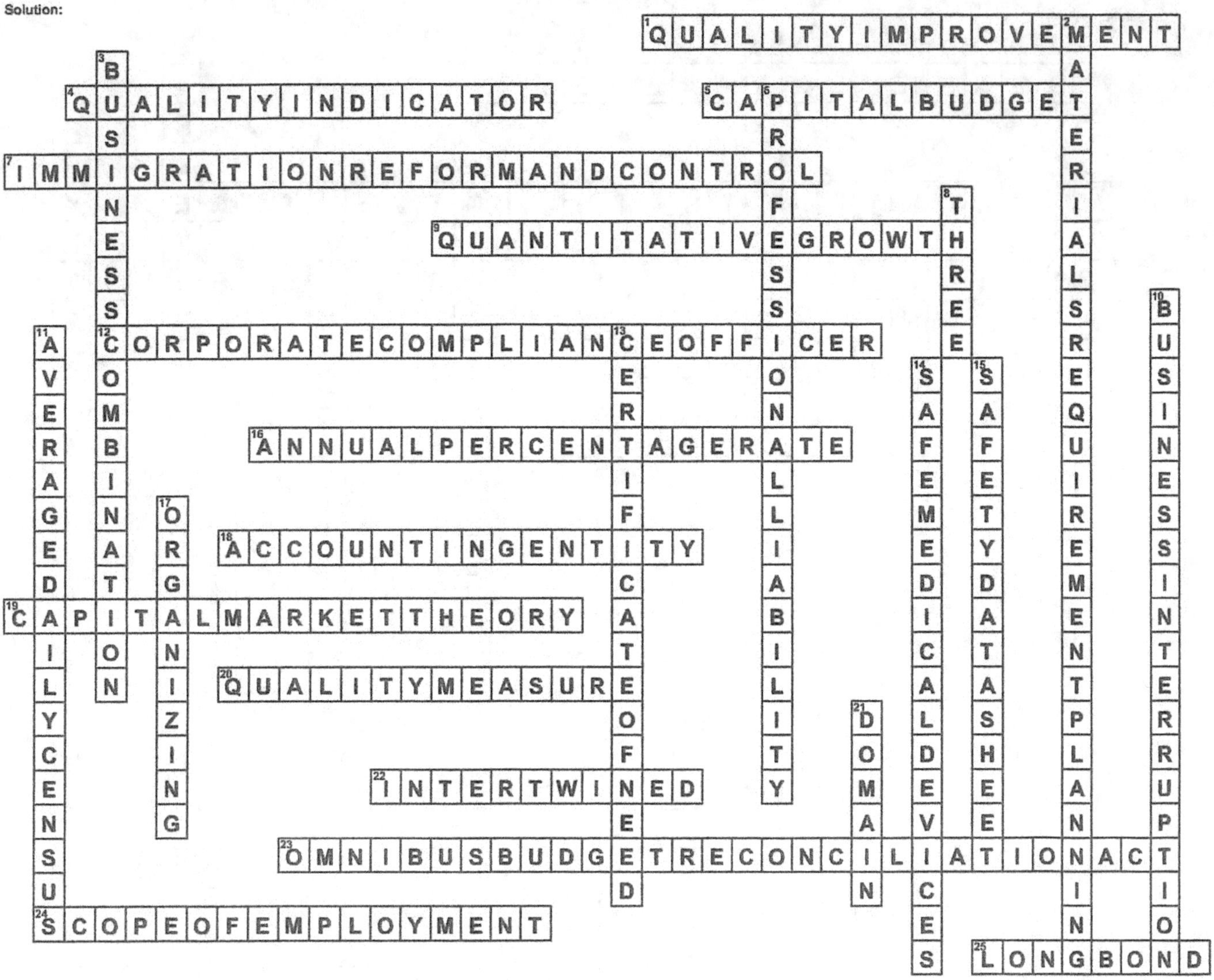

1 QUALITYIMPROVEMENT
2 MATERIALSREQUIREMENTPLANNING
3 BUSINESSCOMBINATION
4 QUALITYINDICATOR
5 CAPITALBUDGET
6 PROFESSIONALLIABILITY
7 IMMIGRATIONREFORMANDCONTROL
8 THREE
9 QUANTITATIVEGROWTH
10 BUSINESSINTERRUPTION
11 AVERAGEDAILYCENSUS
12 CORPORATECOMPLIANCEOFFICER
13 CERTIFICATEOFNEED
14 SAFEMEDICALDEVICES
15 SAFETYDATASHEET
16 ANNUALPERCENTAGERATE
17 ORGANIZING
18 ACCOUNTINGENTITY
19 CAPITALMARKETTHEORY
20 QUALITYMEASURE
21 DOMAIN
22 INTERTWINED
23 OMNIBUSBUDGETRECONCILIATIONACT
24 SCOPEOFEMPLOYMENT
25 LONGBOND

PUZZLE # 40

Solution:

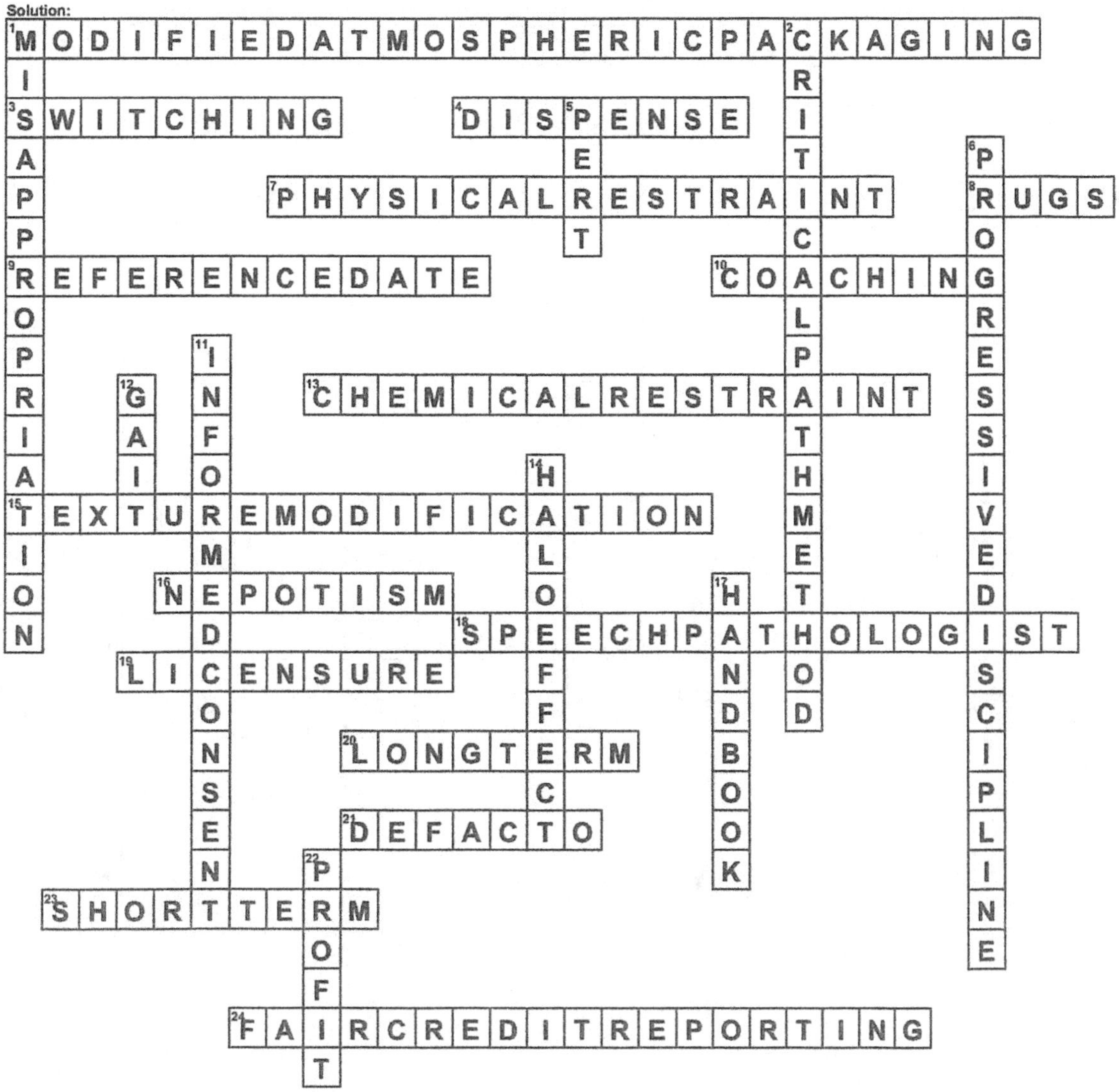
1 MODIFIEDATMOSPHERICPACKAGING
1 MISAPPROPRIATION
2 CRITICALPATHMETHOD
3 SWITCHING
4 DISPENSE
5 PERT
6 PROGRESSIVEDISCIPLINE
7 PHYSICALRESTRAINT
8 RUGS
9 REFERENCEDATE
10 COACHING
11 INFORMEDCONSENT
12 GAIT
13 CHEMICALRESTRAINT
14 HALOEFFECT
15 TEXTUREMODIFICATION
16 NEPOTISM
17 HANDBOOK
18 SPEECHPATHOLOGIST
19 LICENSURE
20 LONGTERM
21 DEFACTO
22 PROFIT
23 SHORTTERM
24 FAIRCREDITREPORTING

PUZZLE # 41

Solution:

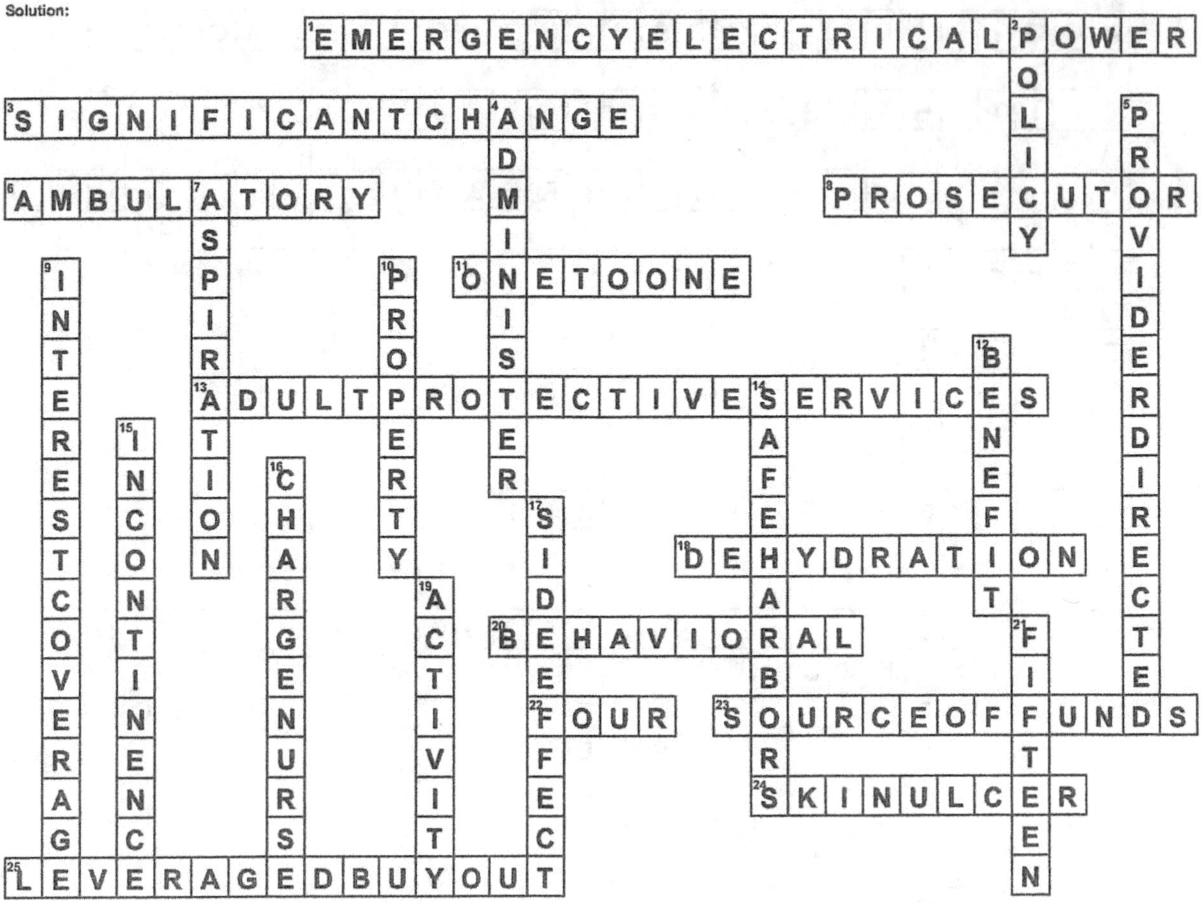

1 EMERGENCYELECTRICALPOWER
2 POLICY
3 SIGNIFICANTCHANGE
4 ADMINISTER
5 PROVIDERDIRECTED
6 AMBULATORY
7 ASPIRATION
8 PROSECUTOR
9 INTERESTCOVERAGE
10 PROPERTY
11 ONETOONE
12 BENEFIT
13 ADULTPROTECTIVESERVICES
14 SAFEHARBOR
15 INCONTINENCE
16 CHARGENURSE
17 SIDEEFFECT
18 DEHYDRATION
19 ACTIVITY
20 BEHAVIORAL
21 FIFTEEN
22 FOUR
23 SOURCEOFFUNDS
24 SKINULCER
25 LEVERAGEDBUYOUT

PUZZLE # 42

Solution:

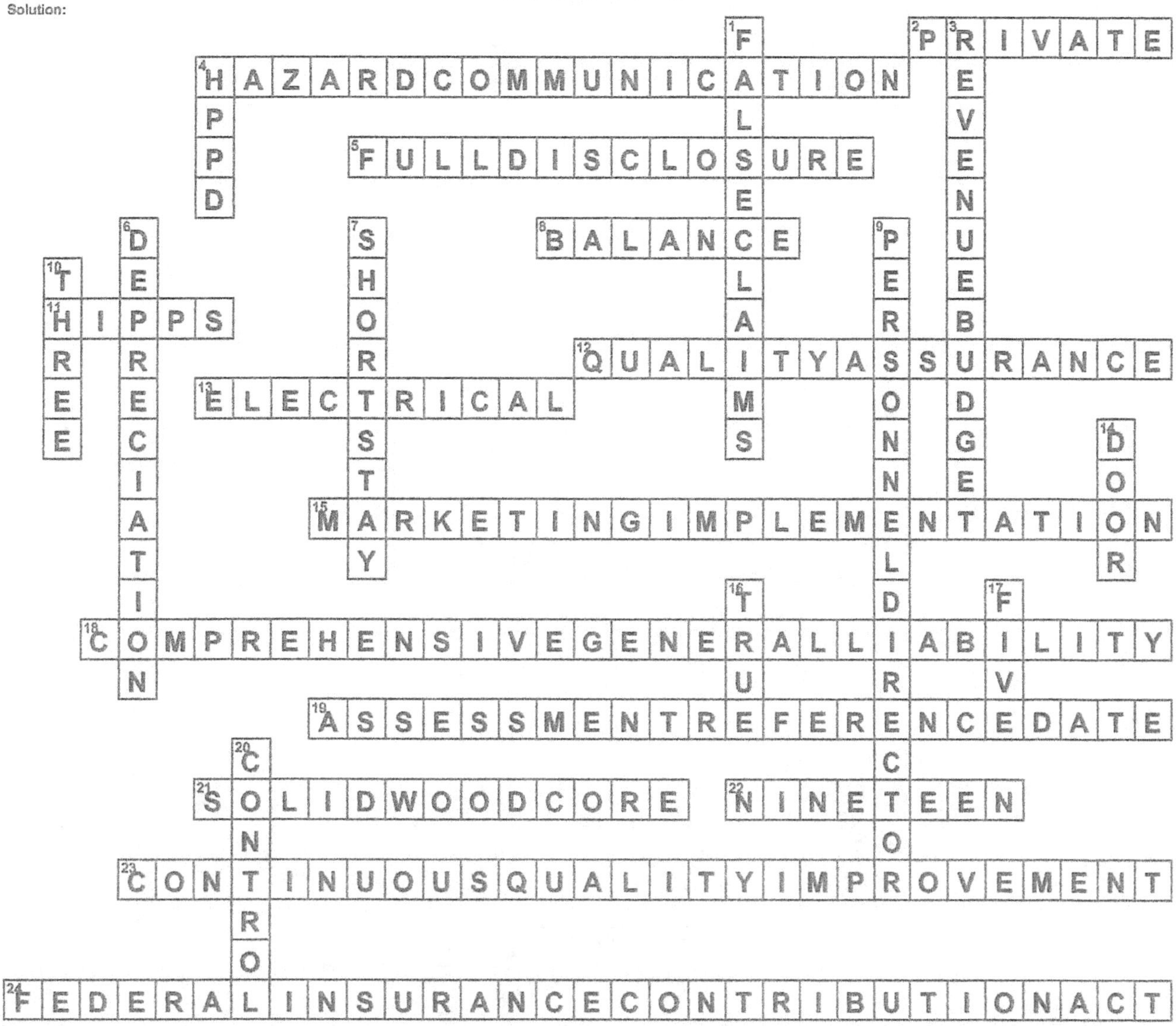

1 FALSECLAIMS
2 PRIVATE
3 REVENUEBUDGET
4 HAZARDCOMMUNICATION
HPPD
5 FULLDISCLOSURE
6 DEPRECIATION
7 SHORTSTAY
8 BALANCE
9 PERSONNELDIRECTO
10 THREE
11 HIPPS
12 QUALITYASSURANCE
13 ELECTRICAL
14 DOOR
15 MARKETINGIMPLEMENTATION
16 TRU
17 FIV
18 COMPREHENSIVEGENERALLIABILITY
19 ASSESSMENTREFERENCEDATE
20 CONTRO
21 SOLIDWOODCORE
22 NINETEEN
23 CONTINUOUSQUALITYIMPROVEMENT
24 FEDERALINSURANCECONTRIBUTIONACT

PUZZLE # 43

Solution:

Across

1. PREFERREDPROVIDERORGANIZATION
5. LOCALHEALTHCOUNCILMOVEMENT
7. LIMITEDLIABILITY
9. MARKETINGSTRATEGY
13. SELECTIVESPECIALIZATION
15. NETPROFITMARGIN
18. CONTROLLEDSUBSTANCE
22. FIXED
23. CERTIFIEDDIETARYMANAGER
24. SIXTYFIVE
25. EMPLOYEERETIREMENTINCOMESECURITY

Down

2. AFFIRMATIVEACTION
3. THIRTYSIX
4. PLANOFCARE
6. INVESTMENTGRADE
8. QUALITYCONTROL
10. AICPA
11. PERCENTILERANK
12. JUNK
14. ONEHUNDREDSIXTY
16. BENCHMARKING
17. SCHEDULEONE
19. ENABLERS
20. FINANCELEASE
21. WAGEMIX

PUZZLE # 44

Solution:

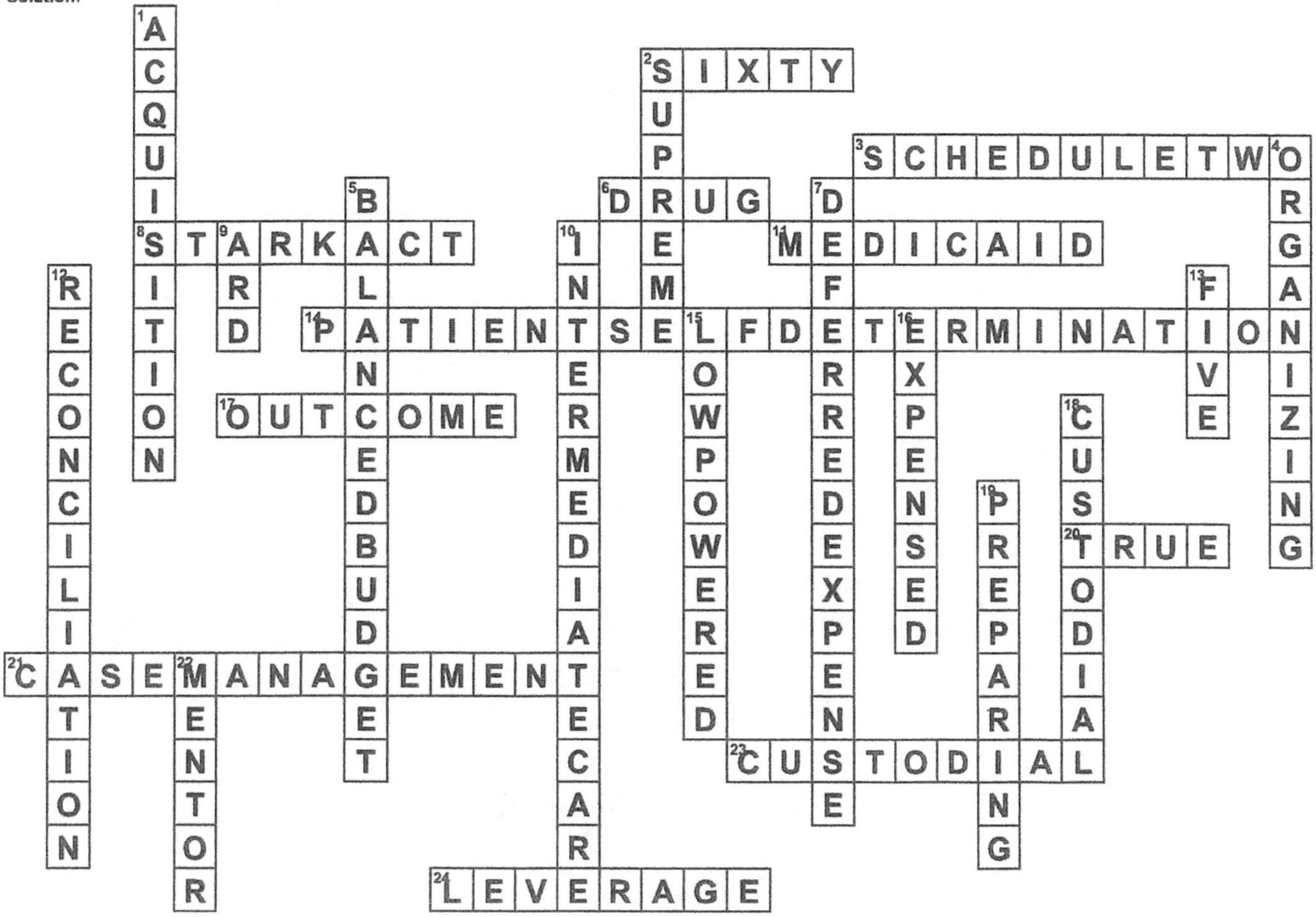

1 ACQUISITION
2 SIXTY
2 SUPREME
3 SCHEDULETWO
4 ORGANIZING
5 BALANCEDBUDGET
6 DRUG
7 DEFERREDEXPENSE
8 STARKACT
9 ARD
10 INTERMEDIATECARE
11 MEDICAID
12 RECONCILIATION
13 FIVE
14 PATIENTSELFDETERMINATION
15 LOWPOWERED
16 EXPENSED
17 OUTCOME
18 CUSTODIAL
19 PREPARING
20 TRUE
21 CASEMANAGEMENT
22 MENTOR
23 CUSTODIAL
24 LEVERAGE

PUZZLE # 45

Solution:

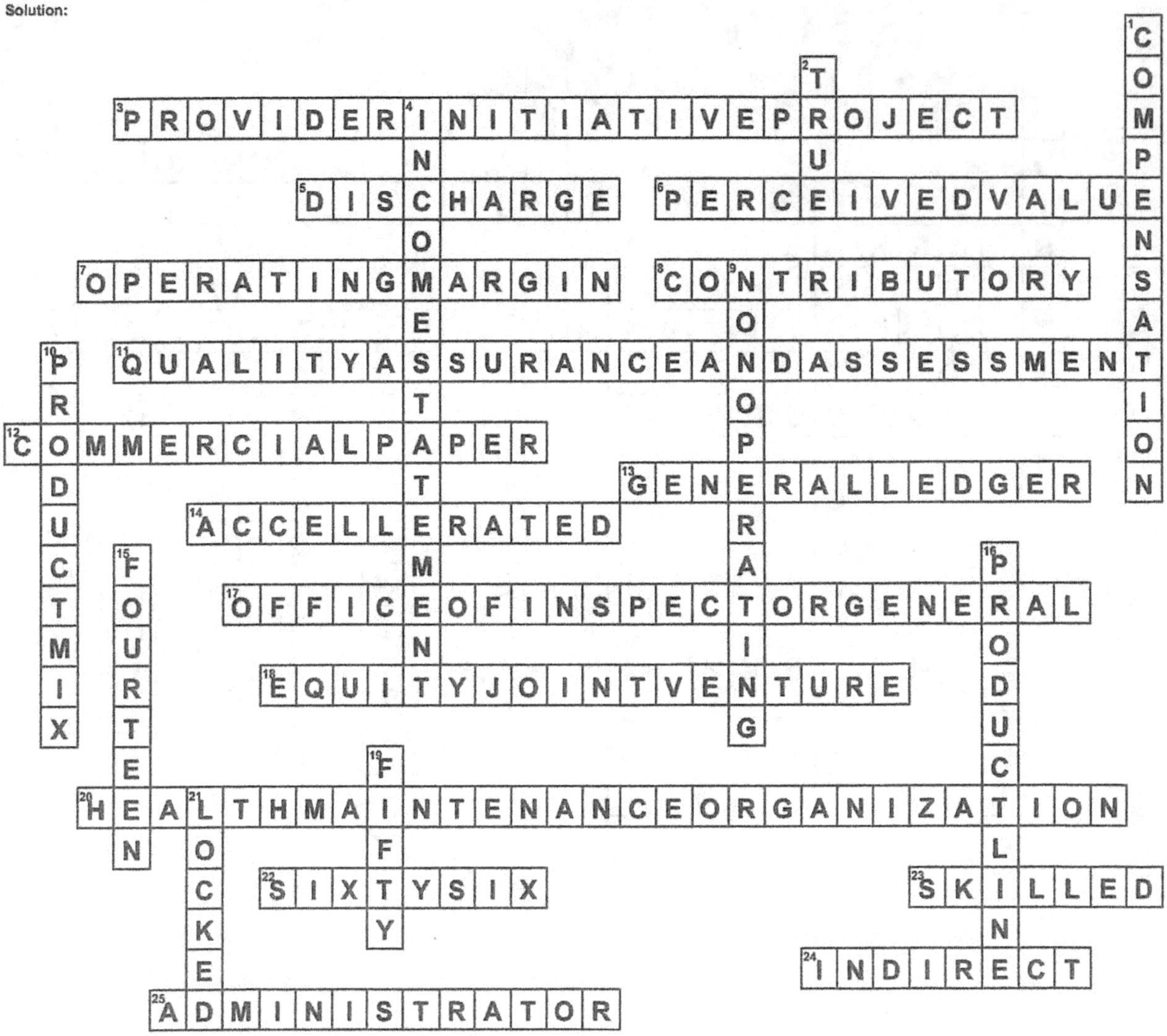

1 COMPENSATION
2 TRUE
3 PROVIDERINITIATIVEPROJECT
4 INCOMESTATEMENT
5 DISCHARGE
6 PERCEIVEDVALUE
7 OPERATINGMARGIN
8 CONTRIBUTORY
9 NONOPERATING
10 PRODUCTMIX
11 QUALITYASSURANCEANDASSESSMENT
12 COMMERCIALPAPER
13 GENERALLEDGER
14 ACCELLERATED
15 FOURTEEN
16 PRODUCTLINE
17 OFFICEOFINSPECTORGENERAL
18 EQUITYJOINTVENTURE
19 FIFTY
20 HEALTHMAINTENANCEORGANIZATION
21 LOCKED
22 SIXTYSIX
23 SKILLED
24 INDIRECT
25 ADMINISTRATOR

PUZZLE # 46

Solution:

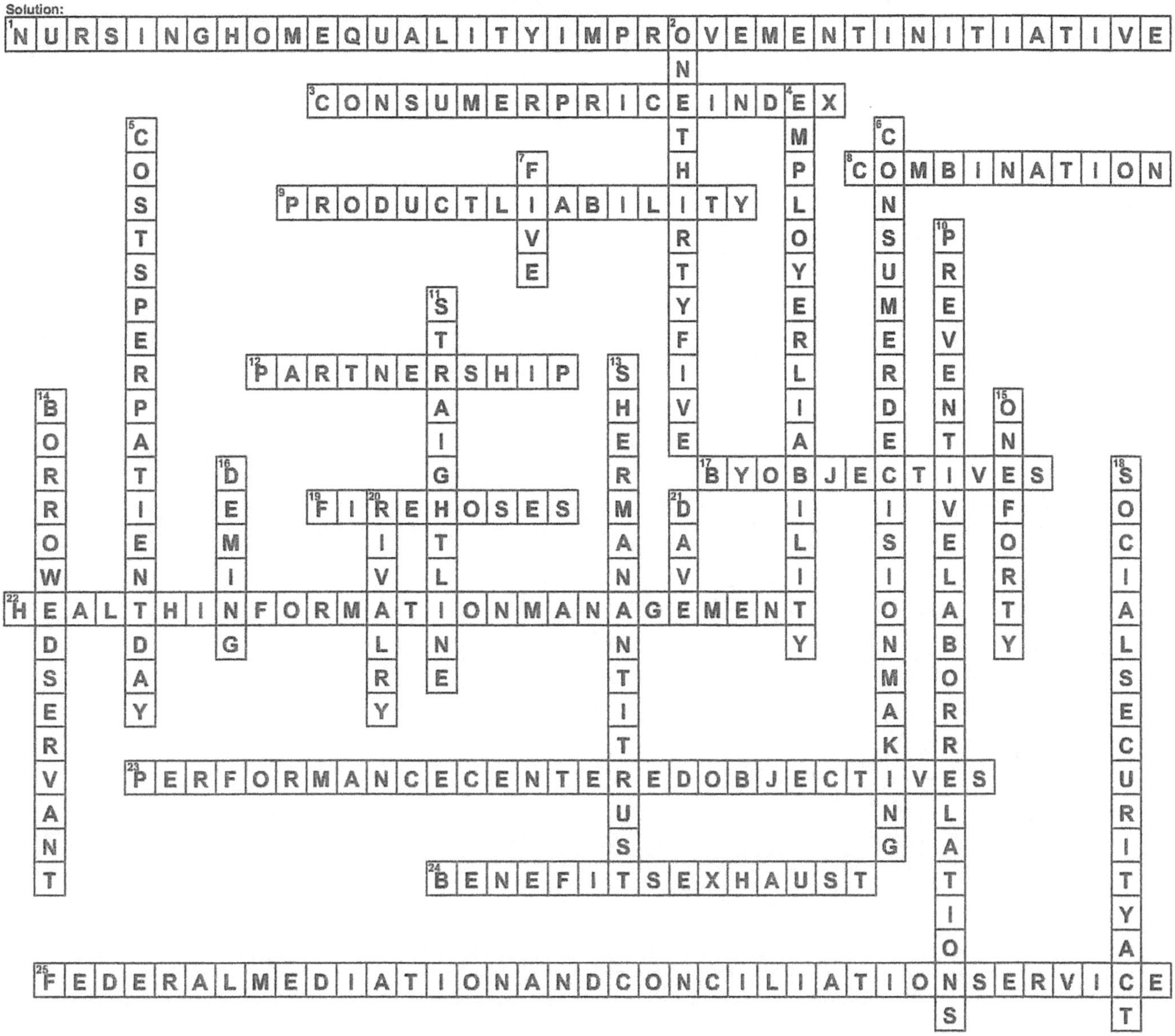
1 NURSINGHOMEQUALITYIMPROVEMENTINITIATIVE
2 ONETHIRTYFIVE
3 CONSUMERPRICEINDEX
4 EMPLOYERLIABILITY
5 COSTSPERPATIENTDAY
6 CONSUMERDECISIONMAKING
7 FIVE
8 COMBINATION
9 PRODUCTLIABILITY
10 PREVENTIVELABORRELATIONS
11 STRAIGHTLINE
12 PARTNERSHIP
13 SHERMANANTITRUST
14 BORROWEDSERVANT
15 ONEFORTY
16 DEMING
17 BYOBJECTIVES
18 SOCIALSECURITYACT
19 FIREHOSES
20 RIVALRY
21 DAV
22 HEALTHINFORMATIONMANAGEMENT
23 PERFORMANCECENTEREDOBJECTIVES
24 BENEFITSEXHAUST
25 FEDERALMEDIATIONANDCONCILIATIONSERVICE

PUZZLE # 47

Solution:

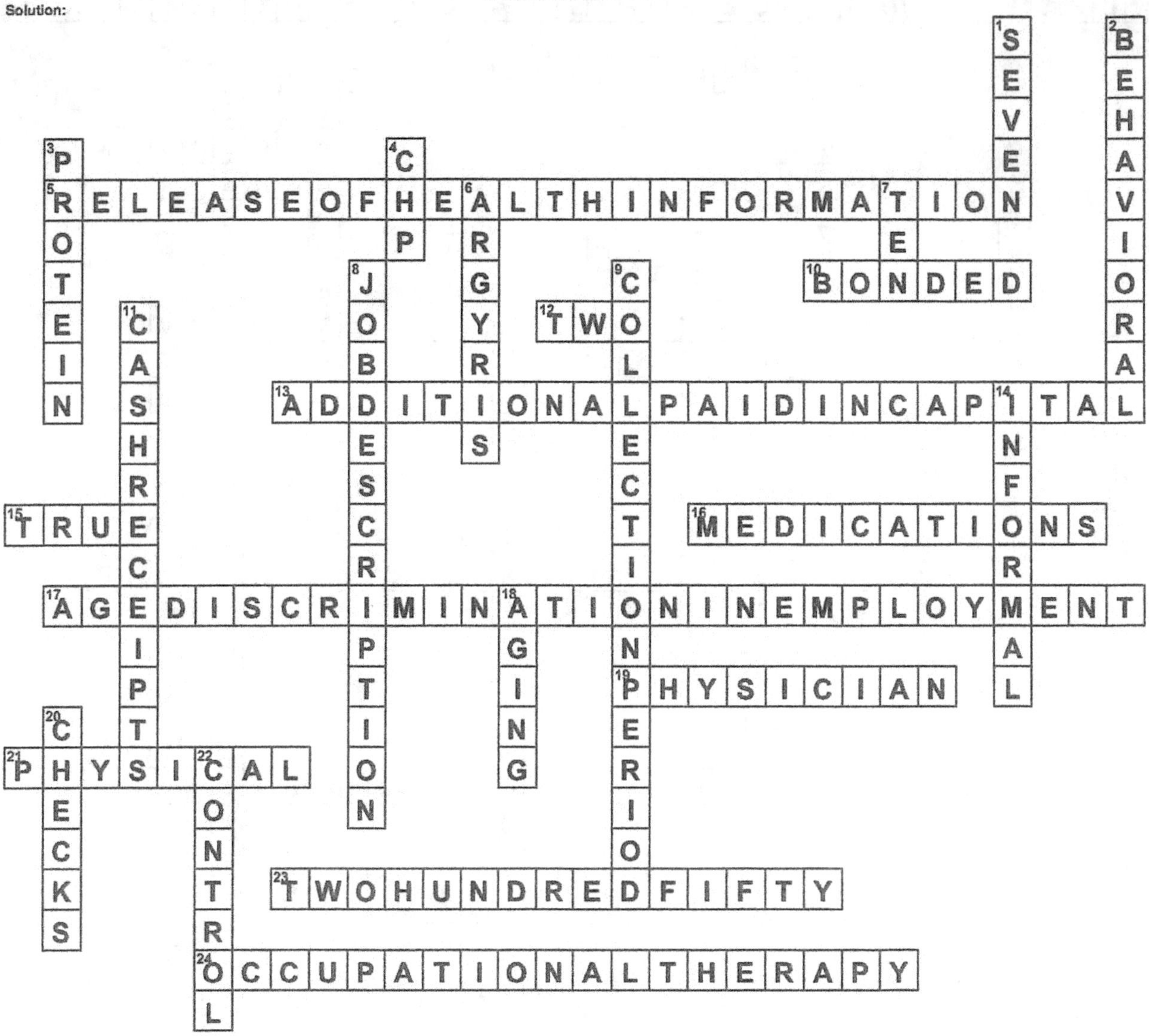
1 SEVEN
2 BEHAVIORAL
3 PROTEIN
4 CHP
5 RELEASEOFHEALTHINFORMATION
6 ARGYRGRIS
7 TE
8 JOBDESCRIPTION
9 COLLECTIONPERIOD
10 BONDED
11 CASHRECEIPT
12 TWO
13 ADDITIONALPAIDINCAPITAL
14 INFORMAL
15 TRUE
16 MEDICATIONS
17 AGEDISCRIMINATIONINEMPLOYMENT
18 AGING
19 PHYSICIAN
20 CHECKS
21 PHYSICAL
22 CONTROL
23 TWOHUNDREDFIFTY
24 OCCUPATIONALTHERAPY

PUZZLE # 48

Solution:

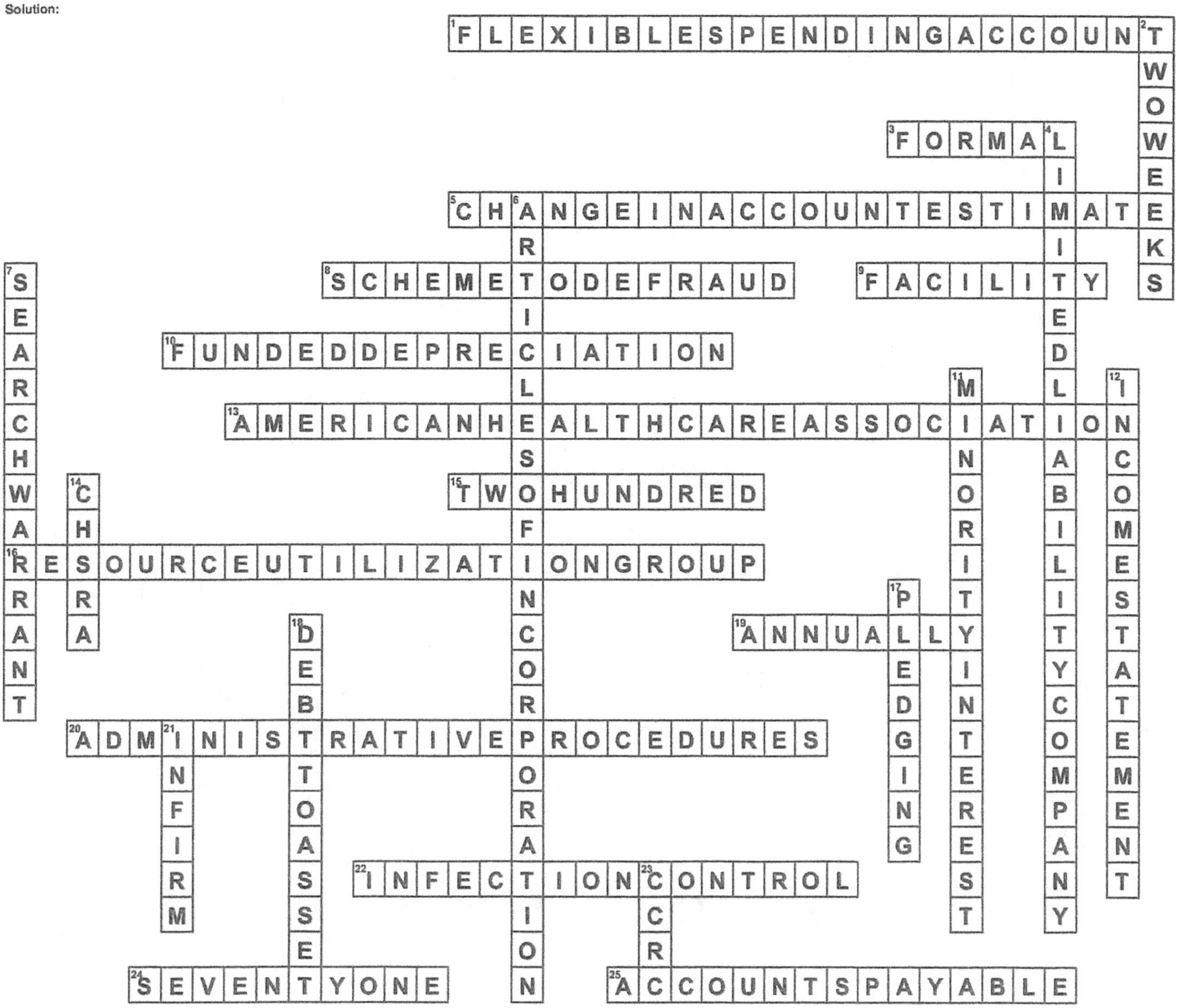

1 FLEXIBLESPENDINGACCOUNT
2 TWOWEEKS
3 FORMAL
4 LIMITEDLIABILITYCOMPANY
5 CHANGEINACCOUNTESTIMATE
6 ARTICLESOFINCORPORATION
7 SEARCHWARRANT
8 SCHEMETODEFRAUD
9 FACILITY
10 FUNDEDDEPRECIATION
11 MINORITYINTEREST
12 INCOMESTATEMENT
13 AMERICANHEALTHCAREASSOCIATION
14 CHSRA
15 TWOHUNDRED
16 RESOURCEUTILIZATIONGROUP
17 PLEDGING
18 DEBTTOASSET
19 ANNUALLY
20 ADMINISTRATIVEPROCEDURES
21 INFIRM
22 INFECTIONCONTROL
23 CCR
24 SEVENTYONE
25 ACCOUNTSPAYABLE

PUZZLE # 49

Solution:

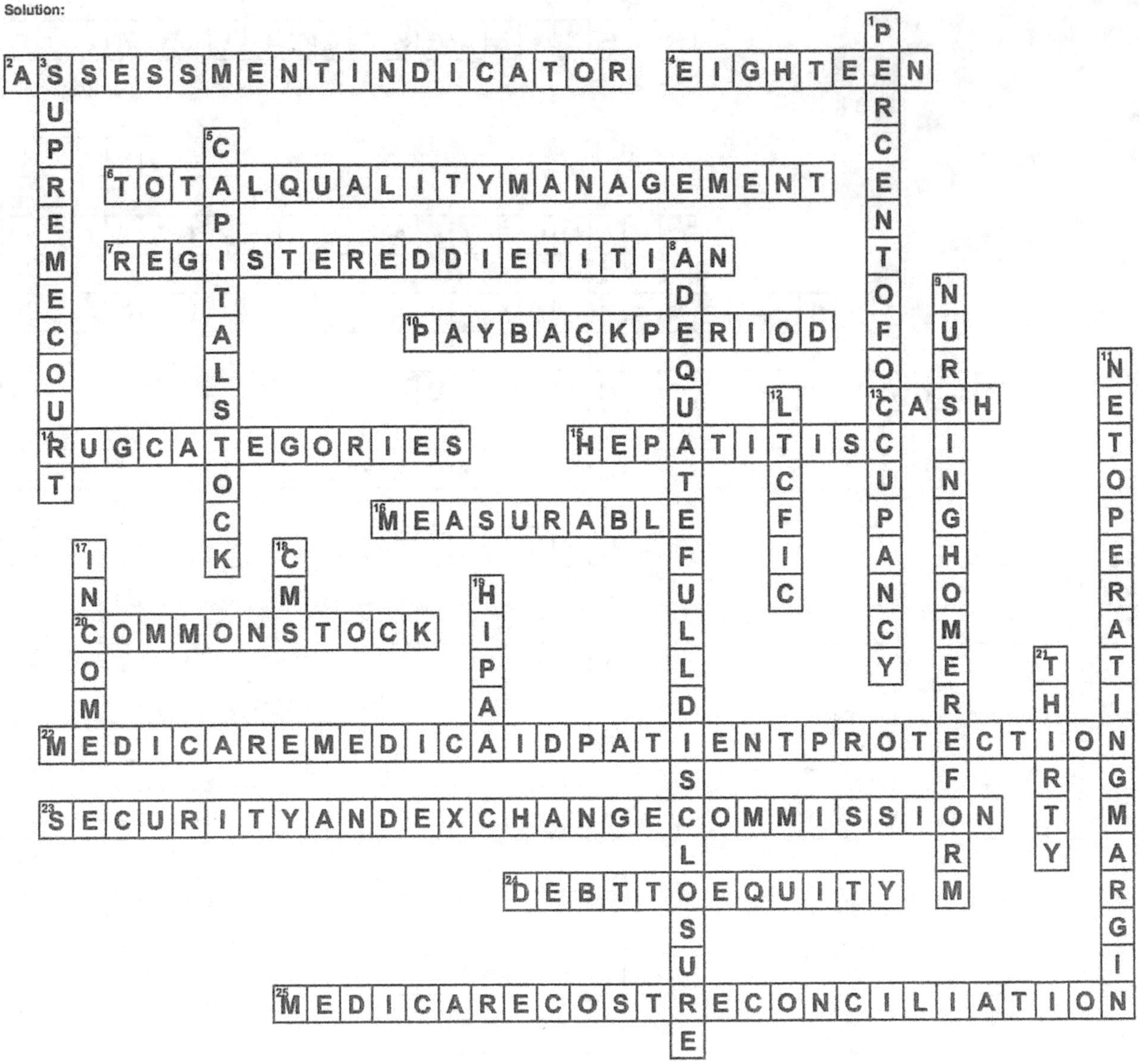
1 PERCENTOFOCCUPANCY
2 ASSESSMENTINDICATOR
3 SUPREMECOURT
4 EIGHTEEN
5 CAPITALSTOCK
6 TOTALQUALITYMANAGEMENT
7 REGISTEREDDIETITIAN
8 ADEQUATEFULLDISCLOSURE
9 NURSINGHOMEREFORM
10 PAYBACKPERIOD
11 NETOPERATINGMARGIN
12 LTCFIC
13 CASH
14 RUGCATEGORIES
15 HEPATITISC
16 MEASURABLE
17 INCOME
18 CMS
19 HIPAA
20 COMMONSTOCK
21 THIRTY
22 MEDICAREMEDICAIDPATIENTPROTECTION
23 SECURITYANDEXCHANGECOMMISSION
24 DEBTTOEQUITY
25 MEDICARECOSTRECONCILIATION

PUZZLE # 50

Solution:

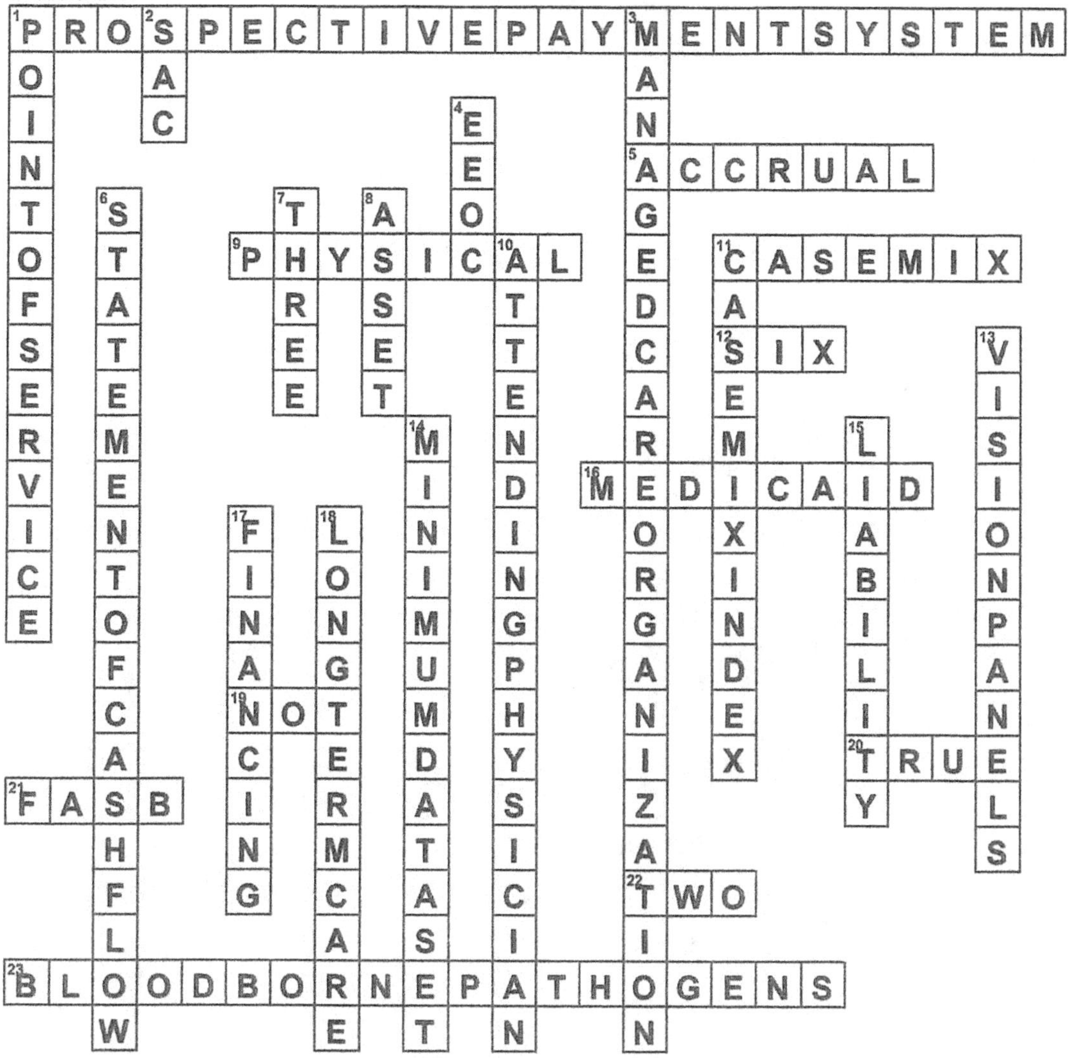

1 PROSPECTIVEPAYMENTSYSTEM
1 POINTOFSERVICE
2 SAC
3 MANAGEDCAREORGANIZATION
4 EEOC
5 ACCRUAL
6 STATEMENTOFCASHFLOW
7 THREE
8 ASSET
9 PHYSICAL
10 ATTENDINGPHYSICIAN
11 CASEMIX
11 CASEMIXINDEX
12 SIX
13 VISIONPANELS
14 MINIMUMDATASET
15 LIABILITY
16 MEDICAID
17 FINANCING
18 LONGTERMCARE
19 NOT
20 TRUE
21 FASB
22 TWO
23 BLOODBORNEPATHOGENS

PUZZLE # 51

Solution:

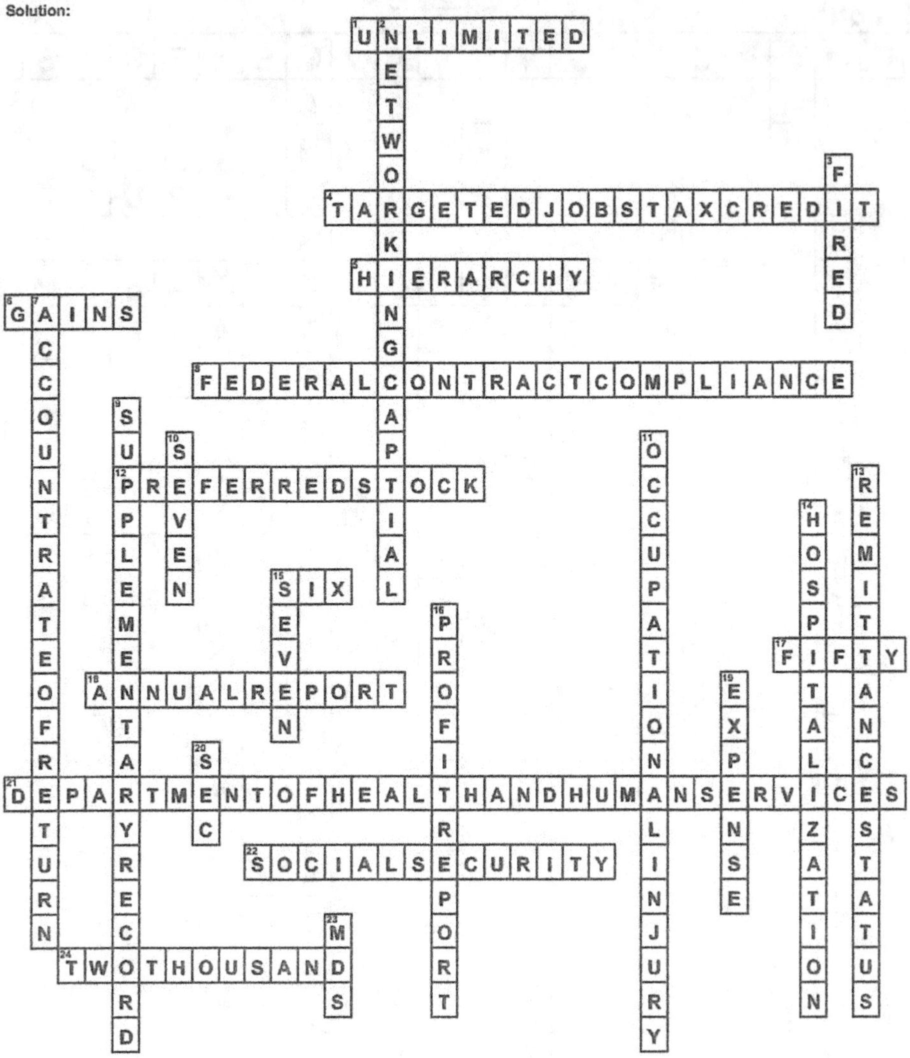
1 UNLIMITED
2 NETWORKINGCAPITAL
3 FIRED
4 TARGETEDJOBSTAXCREDIT
5 HIERARCHY
6 GAINS
7 ACCOUNTRATEOFRETURN
8 FEDERALCONTRACTCOMPLIANCE
9 SUPPLEMENTARYRECORD
10 SEVEN
11 OCCUPATIONALINJURY
12 PREFERREDSTOCK
13 REMITTANCESTATUS
14 HOSPITALIZATION
15 SIX
15 SEVEN
16 PROFITREPORT
17 FIFTY
18 ANNUALREPORT
19 EXPENSE
20 SEC
21 DEPARTMENTOFHEALTHANDHUMANSERVICES
22 SOCIALSECURITY
23 MDS
24 TWOTHOUSAND

PUZZLE # 52

Solution:

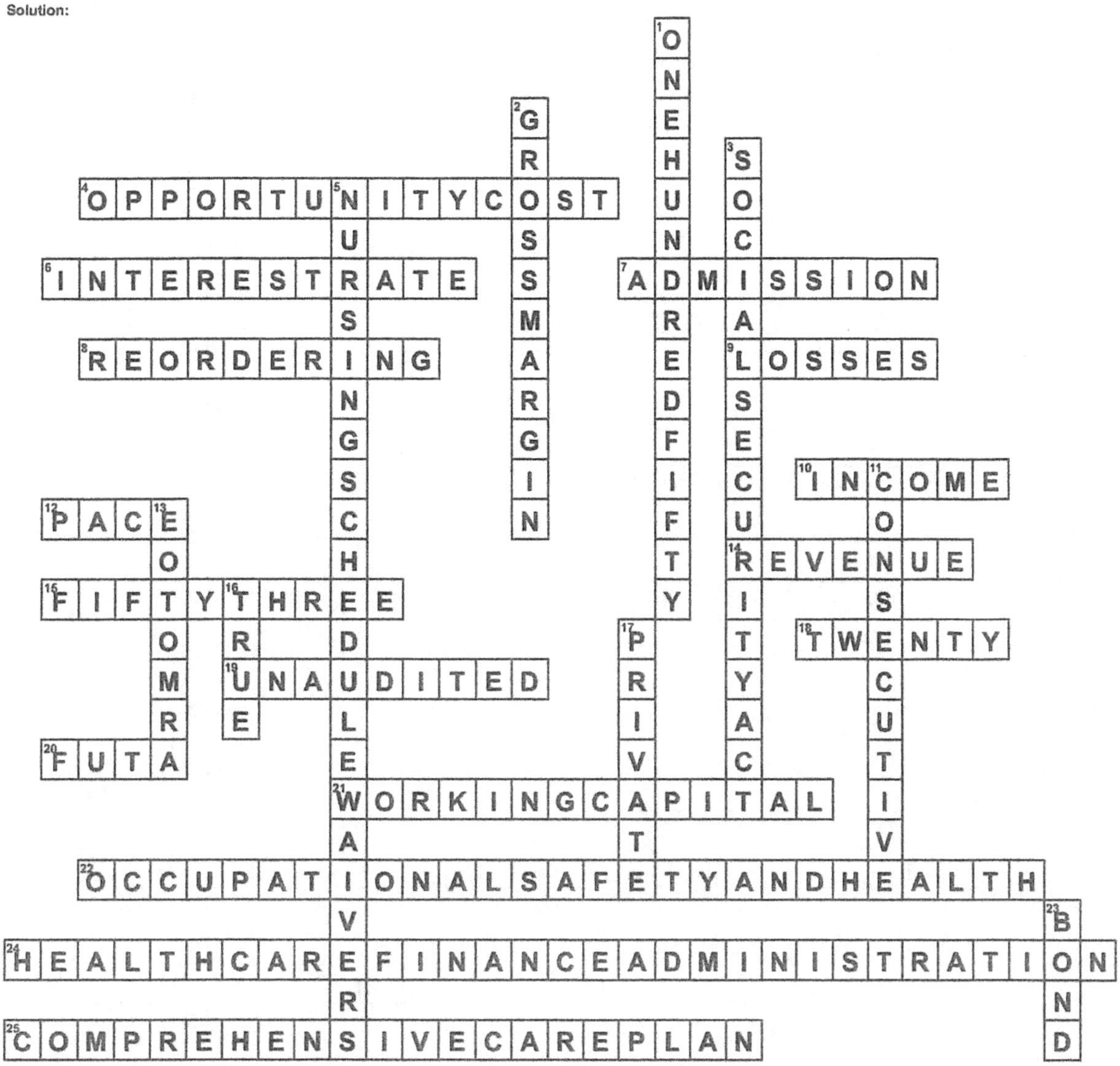

1 ONEHUNDREDFIFTY
2 GROSSMARGIN
3 SOCIALSECURITYACT
4 OPPORTUNITYCOST
5 NURSINGSCHEDULEWAIVER
6 INTERESTRATE
7 ADMISSION
8 REORDERING
9 LOSSES
10 INCOME
11 CONSECUTIVE
12 PACE
13 EOTOMRA
14 REVENUE
15 FIFTYTHREE
16 TRUE
17 PRIVAT
18 TWENTY
19 UNAUDITED
20 FUTA
21 WORKINGCAPITAL
22 OCCUPATIONALSAFETYANDHEALTH
23 BOND
24 HEALTHCAREFINANCEADMINISTRATION
25 COMPREHENSIVECAREPLAN

PUZZLE # 53

Solution:

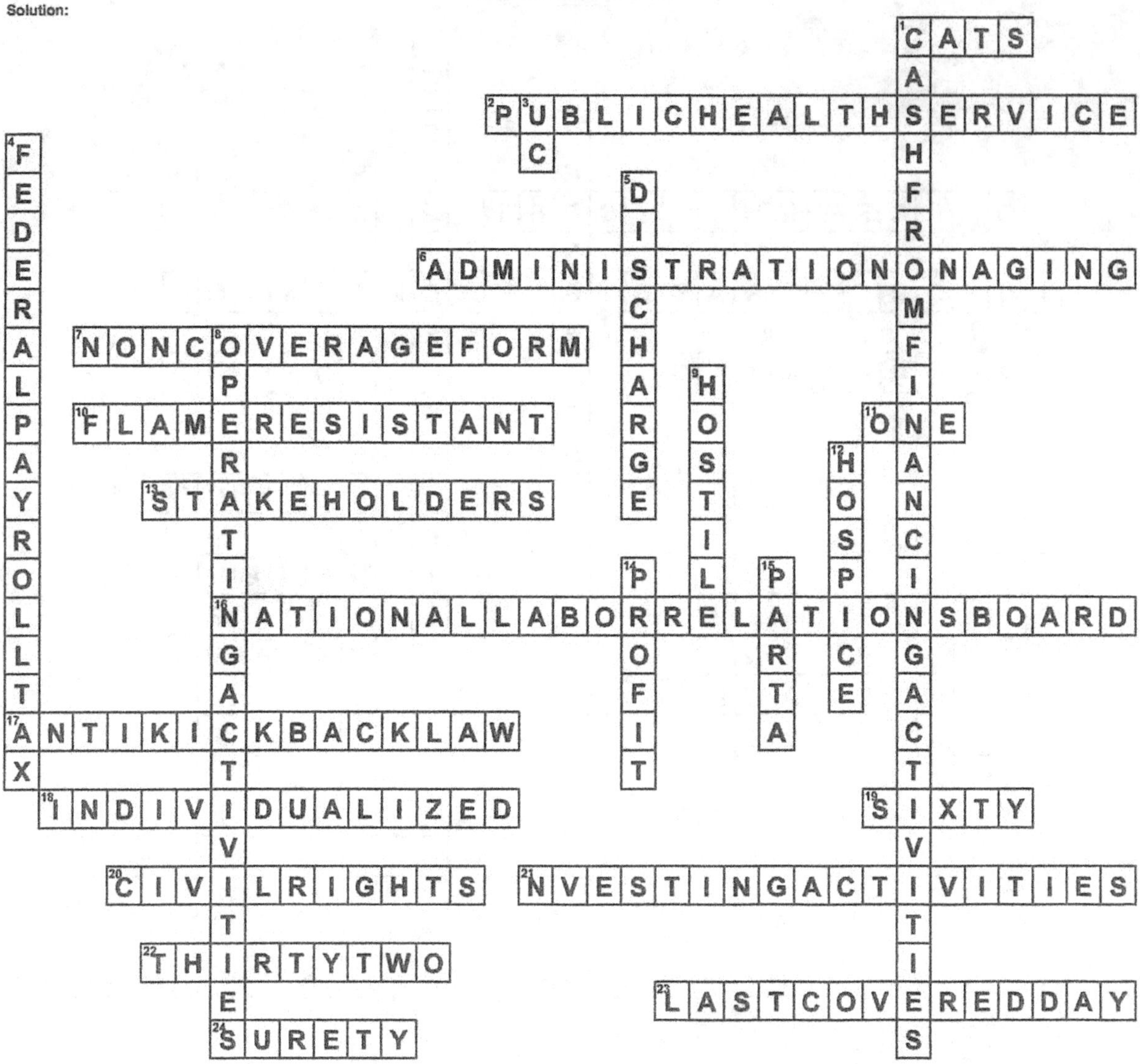

1 CATS
1 CASHFROMFINANCINGACTIVITIES
2 PUBLICHEALTHSERVICE
3 UC
4 FEDERALPAYROLLTAX
5 DISCHARGE
6 ADMINISTRATIONONAGING
7 NONCOVERAGEFORM
8 OPERATINGACTIVITIES
9 HOSTILE
10 FLAMERESISTANT
11 ONE
12 HOSPICE
13 STAKEHOLDERS
14 PROFIT
15 PARTA
16 NATIONALLABORRELATIONSBOARD
17 ANTIKICKBACKLAW
18 INDIVIDUALIZED
19 SIXTY
20 CIVILRIGHTS
21 INVESTINGACTIVITIES
22 THIRTYTWO
23 LASTCOVEREDDAY
24 SURETY

NOTES

NOTES

NOTES

NOTES

www.ingramcontent.com/pod-product-compliance
Lightning Source LLC
Chambersburg PA
CBHW080818180526
45168CB00006B/2499
9781514871362